Brighter Baby

Brighter Baby

by Brenda Adderly, M.H.A.
and
Jay Gordon, M.D.

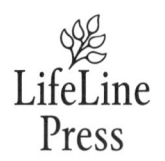

LifeLine Press

Washington, DC

Copyright © 1999 Affinity Communications Corp.

All rights reserved. No part of this publication may be reproduced or transmitted in any form or by any means electronic or mechanical, including photocopy, recording, or any information storage and retrieval system now known or to be invented, without permission in writing from the publisher, except by a reviewer who wishes to quote brief passages in connection with a review written for inclusion in a magazine, newspaper, or broadcast.

Library of Congress Cataloging-in-Publication Data

Adderly, Brenda.
    Brighter baby / by Brenda Adderly and Jay Gordon.
        p.   cm.
    Includes bibliographical references and index.
    ISBN (invalid) 0–89526–393–9.
    1. Massage for infants—Therapeutic use. 2. Sensory stimulation in infants. 3. Infants—Intelligence levels. 4. Infants—Care.
I. Gordon, Jay, 1948– . II. Title.
RJ53.M35A33 1999
649'.122—dc21   98–50803
                                                                                        CIP

Published in the United States by
LifeLine Press
An Eagle Publishing Company
One Massachusetts Avenue NW
Washington, DC 20001

Distributed to the trade by
National Book Network
4720-A Boston Way
Lanham, MD 20706

Printed on acid-free paper.
Manufactured in the United States of America

BOOK DESIGN BY MARJA WALKER
PHOTOS © ROGER FOLEY PHOTOGRAPHY
SET IN BEMBO

10 9 8 7 6 5 4 3 2 1

Books are available in quantity for promotional or premium use. Write to Director of Special Sales, LifeLine Press, One Massachusetts Avenue, NW, Washington, DC 20001, for information on discounts and terms or call (202) 216-0600.

CONTENTS

CHAPTER 1:	Shaping Your Child's Future	1
CHAPTER 2:	The Science of Baby Massage	7
CHAPTER 3:	Ready, Set, Rub: The Basics of Infant Therapeutic Massage	21
CHAPTER 4:	The Experience of Parents	61
CHAPTER 5:	The Mozart Effect: A Link to Baby Intelligence	69
CHAPTER 6:	Brain Development in the Womb and Out	79
CHAPTER 7:	Baby Intelligence and Mother's Diet	83
CHAPTER 8:	Brain Exercises for Your Baby	91

Flashcards:	The Study of Alphabet and Pictorial Images	105
Flashcards:	The Study of Numbers and Languages	133
Intriguing Touch Studies from the Animal Kingdom		145
Glossary		155
References		165
Resources/Addresses		169
Index		171

This book is dedicated to my husband Peter Engel, as well as my twin sons Evan and Connor, who thrive from the magic of baby massage.

— BRENDA ADDERLY

For my wife Meyera who understands attachment parenting better than I do, and for our daughter Simone who has grown into the most wonderful young lady in the world because of this. And of course to my own mother Audrey Gordon. All my love.

— JAY GORDON

CHAPTER 1

Shaping Your Child's Future

The first blush of parenthood is past. You have been blessed with a gurgling, kicking, active baby—one that might keep you up at night, and one that might have your mind focused on the future more than ever before.

That future will not be an entirely random occurrence. You can shape your child's future—and you can do so without drugs, without taking time-consuming parenting classes, without going to any extraordinary expense other than buying this book. All you need to do is to learn how to properly apply and support—perhaps in ways you never thought about before—your own natural inclination to bond with your child and your child's own desire, from her earliest stages of life, for human contact and sensory stimulation.

Through the techniques you will learn in this book, you will be able to raise a healthier, happier child. Most important of all, you can raise a *brighter baby*.

Not only is this possible, increasingly science is teaching us that active, loving parental involvement in a child's first few years is essential. This is the time when a child's brain is "wired" and her ability to learn established.

Miss helping your child during this vital period, and random nature will take its course.

Take an active role in developing your child's mind, and you can grant her the gift of a brain that has a greater capacity for learning and shape a character that is happier and better able to answer the challenges of life.

Do you want your child to have a higher IQ?

Do you want her to have an appreciation, perhaps even an early genius, for music?

Do you want your child to be gifted in mathematics?

Would you like your child to have the gift of picking up languages easily?

Do you want to improve your child's powers of concentration and conceptual thinking?

Would you like a greater assurance that your child will be healthy, happy, and well-adjusted?

> Infant Therapeutic Massage has proven that it can dramatically improve an infant's test scores on every available scale of alertness, good health, and potential IQ development.

You can do all these things. This book will show you how.

First, we'll show how the breakthrough treatment of Infant Therapeutic Massage has proven—especially with babies most at-risk, those born prematurely—that it can dramatically improve an infant's test scores on every available scale of alertness, good health, and potential IQ development.

Second, we'll show you what you can do *before* your baby is born to improve her chances of success. We'll talk about the Mozart Effect, early exposure to foreign languages, and proper nutrition to give your baby the best possible head start.

Finally, we'll close with suggested "Brain Exercises" to help your baby begin developing the skills and intellectual capacity to excell at anything she sets her mind to do.

It's all a matter of stimulating your child's capacity to learn. From the moment of conception your baby has every genetic gift you can provide. After that, it's up to you to nurture those gifts and help your child develop them.

Some of this development takes place *in utero*. If you're reading this while pregnant, there are things you can do *now*, which we will show you, to assist your baby's development.

But much is left to be done post-partum, and one of the most important, but neglected, tools is the gift of loving hands that take over when the comfort of the womb is abandoned.

Therapeutic baby massage, as we will show, can have a dramatic beneficial effect for your baby. Infant Therapeutic Massage has been shown to improve sleeping and eating habits. It reduces tension in babies easily frustrated by their inability to communicate except through tears and wails. It makes for happier, calmer children, enhances communication between parent and child, and offers other physical and intellectual benefits for a child's development.

Some of these benefits involve more complex social skills. It has been shown, for instance, that infants and pre-school children who have affectionate and caring parents are more likely to show empathy and comfort distressed children.

But most important of all, Infant Therapeutic Massage can improve your child's intellectual development—both her ability to grasp complex ideas and her ability to understand people.

Touch and Good Parenting

Our skin is the largest of all our organ systems, comprising about eighteen square feet when we are an adult, weighing about eight pounds, and studded with more than five million nerve endings or receptors.

At eight weeks old, human embryos less than an inch long have already begun to develop skin sensitivity, which continues to increase during the next seven weeks until every part of the body except the top and back of the head, is highly sensitive to touch.

Indeed, Dr. Ashley Montagu, author of *Touching: The Human Significance of the Skin,* asserts that the uterine contractions of labor are the "beginning caresses" of the new infant, and he advocates the continuation of caressing for a considerable time after birth. He is joined by French obstetrician-gynecologist Frederick Leboyer, who advocates that newborns receive a deep, slow massage of their backs, once pressed so closely against the "embrace of the womb."

But whatever the specific recommendations, all the research and techniques related to touch and massage therapy are based on the fact that those five million nerve endings in our skin are there for a reason. Men and women, babies and children, are meant to be touched, to respond to touch. It is one of the vital links between, for example, a mother and child. It is the foundation of parent-child "bonding."

The process of physical bonding begins as soon as a baby is placed in a mother's arms, and it begins with touching. Typically, a mother begins to explore the baby's cheeks and fingers with her fingertips. Within the next ten minutes, she strokes the child with the palm of her hand, eventually holding the baby in a close embrace. She begins talking to the child, calling him by name, immediately linking touch, personhood, and learning.

Scientists involved in touch therapy research believe there are at least two interconnected reasons why massage works so well. Part of the answer lies in the principal of *vis medicatris naturae*, "the body heals itself." Massage prompts the body to release natural healing agents—specifically, *endorphins*, the body's natural painkillers—and it also increases the levels of *serotonin*, a natural antidepressant.

Another contributor is that humans are "hardwired" from birth to benefit from being touched. As such, kneading the muscles stimulates the vagus nerve, which is one of the body's largest and most complex nerve systems. The vagus nerve has two major branches: one links the brain to the heart, and relates to speech, alertness, relaxation, and stress hormones; the other links the brain to the gastrointestinal tract, and relates to digestion and hormones such as insulin, which promote food absorption.

But we can also rely to a certain extent on common sense. As every mother who has ever stroked a fractious child to calmness, or hugged a bruised and wailing child to "make it better" knows, a mother who holds and touches her child calms the child through the expression of her love. The baby's stress will decline (this can be easily measured in the reduction of the baby's cortisol levels), and it will be more aware and alert, and, naturally, happier.

This is the way nature intended it to be, for we know that if a mother has, or develops, an aversion to contact with her child during the first three months of its life, both the mother and the infant will suffer emotional problems. Research indicates that a disproportionate number of abused and neglected children are raised by mothers who have an aversion to close body contact.

Further, we know that infants actively seek out the stimulation necessary for the growth and maturation of their sensorimotor, perceptual, and cognitive processes. For infants, the desire for stimulation is a drive, not unlike hunger, and if an infant does not receive stimulation, she suffers. Touch and massage is one of the key tools to providing an infant with the attention she needs.

While this would seem commonsensical, it actually cuts against the grain of many theories of pediatrics, which, though outdated, still have currency with many parents and some doctors.

The giant among these theorists was Dr. Luther E. Holt, a Columbia University professor of pediatrics who wrote at the end of the nineteenth century. Dr. Holt advised that babies should never be picked up no matter how much they cried.

Holt's ideas were reinforced by another giant in the field of psychology, Dr. John Watson, who believed that holding babies only made them psychologically soft and prone to "invalidism," or what we might call hypochondria, as they grew older. Extending this into child rearing, Watson advised that parents never hug or kiss their children or hold them on their laps—all prohibitions quite contrary to most mothers' natural instincts. Any show of love or close physical contact spoiled children and made them too dependent on their parents, which, in the long run, would make them too dependent on the affection of others, or so said Watson.

> Infant Therapeutic Massage can improve your child's intellectual development—both her ability to grasp complex ideas and her ability to understand people.

But what we now know is that touch, far from retarding a person's development, is essential to it, heightening perception and awareness, increasing the ability to learn, improving health, and increasing empathy. But there is something else to remember as well. The early parent-child relationship, while glorious, can also be full of stress. Sleep-deprivation and post-partum depression (which can afflict both men and women) are common parental complaints. But baby massage can help because of the mutual benefits, physical and psychological, of simple touch.

Most people love to be massaged, and babies are no exception. They grin and chortle as you stroke them, kick their legs and gurgle, and clench their tiny hands in apparent delight. They love both the sensation and the attention. Their happiness can be its own reward, but it also feeds a parent's happiness, and can have other residual beneficial effects that parents can notice and employ immediately.

If your baby is crying, massage will often stop the tears. If your baby is awake when both of you ought to be sleeping, massage will often do the trick. A friend says that when her twins become fractious at mealtime and won't eat properly, distracting each other and generally acting up, her husband simply massages their feet and they settle down in no time and get on with their suppers.

Author Amelia Auckett, former nurse-in-charge at the Maternal and Child Health Centers in the Shire of Flinders, Australia, suggests massage can even help in the weaning process. She cites the case of one mother who had difficulty weaning her baby and began giving her nine-month-old baby a massage at his usual time for feeding. Then she gave him a bottle, which he accepted. The mother continued this practice for one month until the baby began to enjoy his 7 PM bottle and went to sleep afterward.

By studying the research, we have been able to identify ten major ways that pediatric massage helps babies and children to be smarter, stronger, and happier. It:

- ❖ offers crucial sensory stimulation
- ❖ enhances calmness and self-assurance
- ❖ heightens feelings of comfort and joy
- ❖ promotes truly restful sleep
- ❖ stimulates appetite and digestion
- ❖ improves breathing
- ❖ benefits skin and muscle tone
- ❖ improves muscular coordination and physical development
- ❖ promotes a better body image and understanding
- ❖ offers an alternative to more invasive therapies (like drugs)

In the next chapter, we'll look at the scientific research behind some of these benefits.

CHAPTER 2

The Science of Baby Massage

The evidence for the benefits of baby massage—drawn especially from the evidence relating to the care of the most needy, premature babies—is startling.

It used to be thought that premature babies were so fragile that touching them should be avoided, because their tiny bodies and nervous systems would be unable to absorb the shock of physical contact.

Now we know better. "Preemies" show remarkable improvement—dramatic gains in growth and health—when treated to careful infant massage. Just as important, the premature babies' intellectual development shows similar positive strides. The evidence that premature babies given regular "tactile stimulation" score higher on measures of infant mental development has been accumulating in studies that date back to at least the 1960s.

Some of the initial evidence came from observant doctors and nurses who noted the effect of the *absence* of touch on babies. One of the first of these was René Spitz, an obstetrician at a hospital for abandoned babies and those of young mothers (often minors) in prison. Dr. Spitz noticed that even though the infants were well-fed and cared for in sanitary conditions, a great many of them died of what later came to be called the "failure-to-thrive" syndrome. While vacationing in Mexico, Dr. Spitz visited an orphanage that had much less sanitary conditions than his own hospital, yet the babies were thriving. Why? Dr. Spitz concluded it was because village women came in daily to hold and rock the babies, to talk and sing to them, while children in his own hospital were dying of "touch starvation." In other words, the best medical care in the world could not compensate for the lack of parental love. Dr. Spitz's now-classic observations spawned a number of studies regarding the importance of touch for infants and resulted in babies in hospital nurseries being held more frequently. They also hastened the trend toward the use of foster homes rather than orphanages, and of earlier placement ages for adoption.

One of the most dramatic studies about the beneficial effects of touch occurred in the late 1970s, when a group of nurses initiated a program of light massage and gentle rocking for premature babies. Not only did the infants's cardiac response to tactile stimuli resemble that of a healthy, full-term infant, but the massaged babies began to visually explore their world in a way that other premature babies did not. Moreover, the massaged babies had accelerated ability to recognize objects they touched. By six months, their visual memory skills were as well developed as those of full-term babies. That was exciting enough, but what has made this discovery even more important is that visual recognition memory tests are now known as an accurate predictor of childhood IQ scores. This was one of the first indications that baby massage could effect IQ.

Another breakthrough study occurred in 1977, when, for her doctoral research, Ruth Dianne Rice, nurse, psychologist, and specialist in early child development, created a structured, sequential infant stroking and massage technique. Known as Rice Infant Sensorimotor Stimulation (RISS), the technique specified variations in pressure, finger-tip rotation, and rhythm. The massage began at the head, and continued to the arms, chest, back, and legs. Each stroke was repeated three times; nothing was left to chance.

Rice taught the procedure to nurses, who taught the technique to fifteen mothers to use with their babies. A control group of fourteen mothers of premature babies was taught usual newborn care, but no massage.

The "massage mothers" administered the massage for fifteen minutes, four times a day. The massage was followed by five minutes of rocking, holding, and cuddling.

After four months, the infants' neurological development, weight, length, head circumference, and mental and motor development were assessed by a

THE SCIENCE OF BABY MASSAGE

pediatrician, a psychologist, and a pediatric nurse and compared to the control group. Dr. Rice concluded that "the experimental infants made significant gains in neurological development... and in mental development" and that "the findings indicate that the early and systematic stimulation provided by mothers can enhance development of premature infants." Dr. Rice and her colleagues also suggested that, based on animal studies, it was likely that infant massage probably achieved this effect for premature babies by:

❖ speeding up the growth of the brain and nervous system by increasing myelination, a process of building up a protective coating around nerve fibers;
❖ increasing the development of dendritic processes (message-receiving parts of the brain);
❖ raising the Nissl substance (protein bodies) in brain cells, which further augments the dendritic process;
❖ promoting increased cellular activity and endocrine functions by increasing the output of the hypothalamus, which in turn, causes faster weight gain by increasing the output of somotrophin, a growth hormone.

In the mid-1980s, a team of researchers did a "meta-analysis" (review and analysis) of nineteen stimulation studies done on pre-term infants and found that more than seventy percent of the preemies who received regular touch therapy did better—in weight gain, motor/reflex performance, and visual/auditory alertness—than control groups not receiving similar stimulation.

Similar effects were found in studies that branched out from studying premature babies to studying the effect of touch on infants generally.

Baby Yoga

Yoga classes for babies are a growing trend in gyms and alternative health clinics across the country, providing another way to create a special bond between you and your baby.

Yoga for babies does not, obviously, concentrate on the meditation aspect of yoga, but focuses on bringing mother and child together through exercise. Baby yoga classes teach gentle yoga positions and stretches that will be both stimulating and relaxing for your baby. Sometimes moms participate by holding the babies on their laps or by performing stretching exercises with their babies.

Babies participating in yoga are said to be more physically adept and emotionally secure.

Marshall Klaus and John Kennell, pediatric professors at Case Western Reserve University in Cleveland, Ohio, reviewed seventeen such studies, covering the 1970s and 1980s, and concluded that early touching—simple caressing of a child—led to higher reading scores, richer speech patterns, and significantly higher IQs.

One of the pivotal studies on infant massage happened in 1984—pivotal, because it involved two medical establishments of sterling reputation: the Department of Pediatrics at the University of Miami Medical School, and the Department of Pharmacology at Duke University.

The study focused on the effects of "tactile/kinesthetic stimulation" on forty preterm babies in a neonatal intensive care unit. The babies chosen had to be free of any congenital heart or other physical malformations, have no gastrointestinal or central nervous system problems, and not be born to mothers who were drug addicted. Once the preemies were stable—that is, they were gaining weight and no longer needed additional oxygen or intravenous feedings—they were admitted to a transitional or "grower" nursery.

> *So vibrant is the power of touch that the massage-giver enjoys as many significant health benefits as the massage recipient.*

The forty babies were then assigned to either a "stimulation" or a "control" group, with twenty babies in each group, matched on a number of characteristics, including age, birth weight and weight at the onset of the study, birth length, head size, and other measures to ensure the babies did not differ in physical or behavioral maturity. All the babies were in "isolettes"—the incubators for premature babies—and bottle-fed. But the twenty babies in the control group did not receive the specific tactile and kinesthetic—that is, muscular and movement-oriented—stimulation that the other twenty babies did.

For ten days, the twenty infants in the stimulation group received "stimulation" for three fifteen-minute periods. The stimulation was broken down into two parts: "tactile stimulation," with the baby lying prone (tummy down) and stroked through the isolette portholes in a specific head-to-toe sequence, and "kinesthetic stimulation," with the baby on her back and given a series of flexion/extension movements for her arms and legs.

Remarkably, babies who were massaged averaged forty-seven percent more weight gain per day than those babies not massaged, even though the babies did not differ on number of feedings per day or average formula intake. Massaged babies were also more alert, active, and responsive, and were healthy enough to be released from the hospital six days earlier than the nonmassaged babies.

In the 1990s the importance of touch and baby massage has been affirmed and awareness heightened by the Department of Pediatrics at the University of Miami School of Medicine, which is the home of the Touch Research Institute, the first center in the world dedicated to basic and applied research on the sense of touch. The institute was founded in 1992 by Tiffany Field, Ph.D., a well-known professor of pediatrics, psychology, and psychiatry.

One of the institute's discoveries in the early 1990s was that the benefits of touch therapy are mutual. So vibrant is the power of touch that the massage-giver enjoys as many significant health benefits as the massage recipient.

For one study, the Institute recruited retiree "grandparent" volunteers and trained them to massage premature, drug-exposed, "failure-to-thrive" newborns, orphans, and abused children. After a month of massage, the infants were more active, their alertness and tracking behaviors improved, they slept better, and they were more sociable and easier to soothe.

But the children were not the only beneficiaries. The retirees showed a dramatic decrease in depression, increased feelings of self-worth, improved sleep patterns, and fewer doctor visits. They reported less anxiety, drank fewer cups of coffee, and their levels of urine cortisol, a stress-related hormone, decreased. In fact, the positive effects on the "grandparents" were greater after giving a massage than after receiving one.

Kangaroo Care

Perhaps an equally remarkable testimony to the power of touch is the growing popularity in neonatal intensive care units of what is known as "Kangaroo Care."

The origin of Kangaroo Care is astonishing. It originated in 1979 in

Bogotá, Colombia, in two doctors' efforts to cut the death rate for premature babies in their country. It began being tested around the world in the 1980s, and is now an established part of many neonatal care units. It is a simple, straightforward approach, based on the basic principle of baby massage—that touch can heal.

Kangaroo Care has a variety of techniques, but it is as easy as a mother holding her diaper-clad baby against her bare breasts, and covering the infant with a blanket for warmth. Depending on its size, the baby may also need booties for extra warmth and a headcap, since the head is one-fifth of the body surface in newborns.

The purpose of Kangaroo Care is to maintain the body temperature of premature infants, but doctors are finding that it has many other benefits as well.

The Stress of Being Born Prematurely

Most studies on Kangaroo Care—like those on baby massage—focus on the premature infants who are most at risk.

Premature infants have a tough time maintaining their body temperature because they lack fat. They have difficulty breathing because their lung tissue is immature. And they have problems getting the nutrition they need because neither their gastrointestinal tract nor their sucking reflex is fully developed.

The third trimester of fetal life is a time when rapid brain development occurs in cortical neurons, the nerve cells on the outer surface of the brain. Dendritic and axonal processes, involving the branching of nerve cells and the nerve cells' ability to send messages throughout the body, are developed, and synaptic contacts that allow the transference of nerve impulses in the brain are established. Because these processes normally occur in the uterus—a warm, dark environment that provides kinesthetic stimulation and hormonal support—there is some concern that while neonatal intensive care units can save lives, their bright, noisy, invasive atmosphere, in which it is difficult for most preemies to sleep, and in which these highly sensitive infants are bombarded by harsh stimuli (so severe that studies have shown that even doctors and nurses can feel "overwhelmed" by the noise, stress, and bright lights), might lead to long-term developmental problems.

Further, research has shown that preterm infants are more likely to cry and be irritable, are often difficult to feed, and might bond less quickly with their parents because of their medical isolation.

How Does Kangaroo Care Affect Babies and Their Mothers?

Kangaroo Care—simply maximizing the skin-to-skin bonding periods enjoyed by mother and child—can have remarkable effects.

Specifically, studies show that Kangaroo Care:

- stabilizes the heart rate
- stabilizes the respiratory rate
- improves the breathing pattern
- improves the dispersion of oxygen throughout the body
- reduces severe bradycardia (heart rate below 100 beats per minute) and apnea (forgetting to breathe)
- almost ends severe tachycardia (heart rate above 180 beats per minute)
- reduces crying; preemies who have benefitted from Kangaroo Care are relaxed and contented and cry less even when returned to their incubator or crib
- contributes to sounder sleep
- often improves feeding vigor and reduces regurgitation
- increases a premature baby's tolerance for the surrounding noise, activity, and medical intervention of a neonatal intensive care unit, making the infant less prone to be startled and less likely to burn much-needed calories in agitation
- shortens hospitalization

> **Touch Your Baby!**
> A mother's touch can have long-lasting positive effects for a baby's development—both physical and mental. But, equally, *not* touching your baby can have detrimental, even harmful, effects. Recent studies have shown that babies who are unloved and untouched have speech and behavior problems, delayed growth, abnormal cognitive and motor skills, and decreased IQ levels.

So great are the results of Kangaroo Care that some authors describe skin-to-skin contact as intensive care without expensive equipment (though of course, it is by no means a replacement for it).

Why and How Does Kangaroo Care Work?

No one is really sure. But we do know that when a preemie is lying on her mother's breast, she can hear the same heartbeat and voice she heard in the womb. It is also an encouragement to nurse. Many preemies don't have the muscle tone or strength to put a thumb to their mouths and may have difficulty retaining a pacifier. Not only do most mothers who practice Kangaroo Care breastfeed, but studies have also shown that they produce more milk.

Another subtle benefit of Kangaroo Care is the position of the baby. While in the womb, babies rest in the "fetal position."

The fetal position turns out to be much more important than most of us realize, and the problem for premature babies is that they are often too weak to maintain it. You can see them lying in an incubator with arms and legs splayed out, losing precious heat by exposing to the air those arteries in the arm, groin, and back of the knee, which are closer to the skin than arteries in other parts of the body.

The fetal position helps maintain and control body heat, but equally as important, it is necessary for the maturation of the infant's nerve cells. Anything that helps that tiny preemie curl up ultimately enhances coordination and development.

Flexion, another name for the fetal position, which is reinforced during any holding, but especially during Kangaroo Care, prevents exposure of arteries to cold air and reduces the surface area from which the infant can lose heat.

One surprising discovery is that in Kangaroo Care, mothers regulate the skin temperatures of their preemies by unconsciously changing the temperature of their breasts. Studies have shown that if a baby held by its mother begins to cool, the temperature in the mother's breasts responds by going up. If a baby becomes too warm, the temperature in the mother's breasts goes down. The mystery of Kangaroo Care is that this phenomenon does not require physical stimulation—that is, the baby's temperature does not actually have to change. A mother holding a baby will also respond physically to the power of suggestion. Someone standing behind her telling her that her baby is getting too cold or too warm can cause the temperature in the mother's breasts to rise or fall. This unconscious regulation is now referred to as "maternal-neonatal thermal synchrony."

The Kangaroo Pouch

However remarkable the results of touch therapy, the means by which they are achieved are simple. Beyond Kangaroo Care, the Rice Infant Sensorimotor Stimulation technique, and other methods, touch therapy can be as easy as using a sling, backpack, or frontpack to carry your child. The important thing is to have skin-to-skin contact, which encourages mother-child and father-child bonding. "Baby-wearing" also has physical benefits, encouraging your child to exercise by flinging her arms and kicking her legs. It offers her the mental stimulation of all the sights and sounds of the outdoor world, and of your smiles, caresses, and speech. It encourages your child to laugh with amazement, surprise, and delight as she sees seagulls or squirrels or products on a supermarket shelf. And, most interesting, it can even help her develop a sense of balance, because the motion offered by baby-wearing stimulates the vestibular apparatus of your child's inner ear. Baby-wearing can also be comforting for a child, and encourage sleep in a fussy baby.

Did you ever think that simply carrying your baby could do so much? It does—and that's the point. It's the little things that matter, and by knowing how they work and what they can achieve, you can create a more stimulating and better nurturing environment for your child. This is especially, and obviously, true when the knowledge of touch is scientifically directed, as with baby massage. How does touch achieve all these benefits—and others we have yet to see? Here are some likely conclusions.

Massage Helps Promote Sleep

In general, massage teaches your baby how to relax. As you continue massage throughout your child's infancy, it will become a skill your child can use for a lifetime.

Before touch was so readily sanctioned, an early, preliminary study showed that placing both full-term and stable preterm infants on specially constructed, continuously oscillating (that is, massaging) waterbeds reduced episodes of apnea (stopped breathing).

Follow-up studies of preterm babies showed that using the waterbeds resulted in longer quiet sleep and decreased irritability when awake. The preemies' movements were smoother and less jerky.

When seven preemies of thirty-three weeks' gestational age were placed on a rocking bed and exposed to heartbeat recordings for two weeks, they developed distinct sleep states earlier and showed a significant increase in quiet sleep than did nine control infants. They also gained more weight and scored higher on general motor maturation.

Although the effect of the heartbeat alone was not separated in this particular piece of research, other studies using only auditory stimulation (a heartbeat recording, white noise, or the mother's voice) were not as definitely positive as those where auditory stimulation was combined with tactile and kinesthetic stimulation.

In one of the few major studies done on full-term babies, massage was given to twenty infants of depressed adolescent mothers. From birth, the infants attended the day care nursery associated with the Touch Research Institute and the University of Miami School of Medicine. The massaged infants were given a fifteen-minute massage between morning feedings, two days a week for six weeks. A comparable control group was rocked instead of massaged.

The massaged babies cried less and had decreased cortisol levels, suggesting that massage may be more effective than rocking for inducing sleep. This coincides with anecdotal reports from weary parents who say that their infant becomes drowsy while being rocked but quickly awakens when the rocking stops.

Another study out of the Touch Research Institute taught depressed adolescent mothers to massage their infants, who showed "disorganized interaction behavior" and disturbed sleep patterns. The infants were given a fifteen-minute massage daily over a two-week period. The results indicate that drowsiness and quiet sleep increased immediately following the massage. In addition, massaged infants made more baby noises, restlessness decreased during mother-infant play and, overall, the mothers found their babies easier to soothe.

Yet another study found that when healthy preschool children ranging

THE SCIENCE OF BABY MASSAGE

in ages from two to four years old received twenty-minute massages twice a week for five weeks, they went to sleep more quickly during nap time.

Massage Stimulates Appetite and Digestion

To grow and be happy—as well as to sleep through the night without crying—a child needs a healthy appetite and a healthy digestive system that is not prone to constipation, gas, and colic. Massage can help.

In one relevant study six premature infants in a South Carolina hospital were given fifteen-minute body rubs from the neck down, and had their arms and legs flexed ("tactile and kinesthetic stimulation") over a period of ten days. The premature babies were not removed from their incubators during the stimulation period. All babies were bottle-fed by nurses.

At the end of the study, the massaged babies were ten percent heavier than the controls. Not only did they take more formula, they were also easier to feed. The controls actually required repeat feedings before they would drink their allotted amount of formula.

Nurses, who did not know the purpose of the study, noted of the control infants: "often spits up," "takes formula poorly," "lethargic." Typical observations of the massaged preemies included: "eager eater," "retains feedings well," and "alert."

> Learning happens over a lifetime, but a child's learning potential might be defined two or three years before she begins school.

Technique, however, is important, because studies show that light stroking is not enough by itself to initiate weight gain.

Improves Breathing

The respiration of full-term infants is characteristically shallow, unstable, and often "inadequate" in the first weeks after birth, but is stimulated reflexively through sucking and physical contact with the mother. Infants who do not suck vigorously do not breathe deeply.

Respiratory problems are the leading cause of death for preemies. Preemies are vulnerable in a variety of ways. The immaturity of their lungs increases their vulnerability to certain diseases, while the flexibility of the immature thoracic cartilage increases their vulnerability to collapse of the chest wall.

Even before the study of touch came into vogue, some early studies showed that various types of touch reduced the risk of infant apnea. In one startling study, preterm infants with respiratory distress syndrome who had nurses gently cradle their heads and touch their abdomens had significantly higher hematocrit levels (ratio of red blood cells to whole blood) and required less oxygen and fewer blood transfusions. They also become more relaxed and slept better.

Massage Improves Muscular Coordination and Physical Development

One of the most obvious benefits of massage is that it stimulates the muscular system, both relaxing and toning muscles. Massage helps with the aches and pains of growing muscles attached to fast growing bones. It reduces stiffness and tightness and keeps growing bodies flexible.

Massage stimulates and activates receptors in the skin, muscles, and joints—assisting your baby in learning to coordinate her muscular movements.

One study of eleven preemies in the neonatal intensive care unit at Buffalo Children's Hospital showed that after ten days of touch therapy the infants had improved general body tone, better head control, greater hand-to-mouth coordination, and were more alert than a group of control preterm infants who received routine nursery care.

One of the most frequently reported developmental delays for preterm infants involves motor functions. Therapeutic infant massage is a proven tool for improving these functions, allowing these babies to move out of intensive care more quickly.

Massage Acts as an Alternative to Drugs

We do *not* mean to imply here that by using massage you should discontinue using any medication your doctor has prescribed; however, it is well-known that relaxation, which massage produces, aids in reducing the effects of certain disorders, often by reducing the amount of stress hormones in the body. In addition, new research shows that tactile stimulation increases the body's production of a substance, which helps produce T-cells responsible for cellular immunity.

Massage Enhances Calmness and Self-Assurance

Stress is a natural part of our adult lives and those of our babies. There is evidence, however, that stress, including prenatal stress (stress hormones in the mother's bloodstream enter the baby's bloodstream), can retard growth of the tibia, the radius, and the metacarpal bones.

We can't stay in stressful situations without damage to our bodies. We need to learn to relax. Touch and massage help babies to regulate their emotional state, moving from stress into calmness.

When we are relaxed, the activity of the sympathetic nervous system decreases and that of the parasympathetic nervous system increases. This means the heart rate, blood pressure, and respiration rates decrease, blood flow to the kidneys increases, and muscles relax. Moreover, we know that massage not only reduces stress, but in infants increases the production of growth hormones.

Smart Child, Strong Child

The fact that massage stimulates growth hormone production in a baby is important in itself, but also in relation to the brain. During a baby's first year of life, her brain more than doubles in volume, reaching almost sixty percent of its adult size. By the time a child is three her brain has essentially stopped growing. Learning, of course, happens over a lifetime, but a child's learning *potential* might be defined two or three years before she begins school. A child's most important tutor is her parents—her sense of self-worth comes from their love, and many of the most important lessons will come from touch.

In the next chapter, we will introduce you to the Adderly Method of Infant Therapeutic Massage. It adopts all of our accumulated knowledge about massage and its links to child development and intelligence. And you can use it for your child starting right now.

CHAPTER 3

Ready, Set, Rub
The Basics of Infant Therapeutic Massage

You've read about all the things massage and touch can do for people of all ages. Now you're ready to discover it firsthand. In this chapter we introduce the Adderly Method of Infant Therapeutic Massage, a type of massage especially developed for infants and young toddlers. First a few basics, and then it will be time to settle down and launch your child toward greater intellectual and physical development.

By the way, don't think that Infant Therapeutic Massage is something only a mother can do. It's also a great way for fathers and other caregivers to participate in their babies' development.

When to Massage

Infant Therapeutic Massage is a gentle and simple process. As with any new health procedure, however, you should check with your physician before beginning. Massage can be done any time of the day and can be repeated throughout the day. Babies like the comfort of a schedule, so once you find what works, stick to it.

When Not to Massage

Do not massage your baby immediately after she has eaten. Give her at least a half hour to digest her food.

Do not massage your baby if she has an infectious disease, or has a skin irritation, infection, or rash. Aside from the hazard of spreading infection or inflaming already irritated skin, sickness often reduces a child's tolerance for touch.

Do not massage a baby with a fever, because massage increases body temperature.

Do not massage where there is a break in the skin, open wound, or cut. Massage stretches the skin and will interfere with the body's natural attempt to bring the skin together and close the wound.

Do not massage over purple or blue bruises.

Do not massage your baby against her will. Massage should be a pleasurable experience for both of you, not a power struggle. Stop the massage if your baby cries and reassure her. Try the massage again when she is more receptive.

> Massage for children with cardiac and circulatory conditions definitely needs physician approval, as the child's circulatory system might not be able to accommodate the increased blood flow a massage supplies.

If your baby is not amenable the first time you try massage, try stroking her gently for about five minutes, possibly along the back. Gradually she will get used to this new kind of touch and allow longer and longer sessions. Then you can add the legs, or the arms, or the tummy, a little at a time until your baby becomes used to a full massage. To further your baby's comfort, you can also give her a toy, or take breaks and simply hold her.

One way to ease your baby into massage is to practice the technique while bathing her. Here soap acts as a natural lubricant, allowing you to glide your hands along to get her accustomed to massage movements.

To Oil or Not to Oil

Massage therapists vary on their opinions about whether or not to use oil for babies. Researchers at the Touch Research Institute have found that full-term infants massaged with oil showed fewer stress behaviors (grimacing and clenched fists) and lower cortisol levels than those massaged without oil.

If you are using a light, firm stroking touch with your newborn, it's unlikely that you will need to use much oil. If your baby has dry skin, the use of oil might be helpful. As your baby gets older and your strokes become a little more firm, oil becomes more useful. Never use so much oil that your hands slip. The goal is for your hands to glide more easily over the baby.

Surprisingly, you should avoid baby oils. Most massage therapists agree that mineral oil—a basis of baby oils—is too heavy and thick for tiny babies, and tends to clog pores, smother skin, and may require scrubbing with soap and water to remove. Some massage therapists don't like using mineral oil because it is a nonorganic product distilled from crude petroleum. They believe that products with a petroleum base should not be used on babies.

When choosing oil, we recommend one formulated especially for baby massage. Also, try to take advantage of the ancient art of aromatherapy. Hippocrates, the father of medicine, said that "the way to health is to have an aromatic bath and scented massage every day." We couldn't agree more.

A Brief History of Massage and Aromatherapy—It's Not Just for Babies

In fact, massage, touch, and aromatherapies, however new they might appear to the layman as tools to achieve good health, have celebrated histories. Massage was practiced by the Chinese as early as 3000 B.C., according to records in the British Museum. The sacred book of the Hindus, the *Ayur-Veda* ("Art of Life"), written around 1800 B.C., also included massage treatments as one of several primary healing practices.

The Secrets of Baby Massage

It has been proven that baby massage:

- relaxes your baby and improves her sleep (and yours!)
- relieves stress and decreases irritability
- improves your baby's digestion and can relieve a colicky baby
- promotes faster weight gain and resistance to infections and diseases
- provides a stimulating environment multiplying neural connections, thereby increasing brain development and intelligence
- promotes muscle development
- reinforces feelings of love and nurturing, making for a happier baby and one who is a joy to be around
- creates a bond and improves communication between you and your baby

The "secret" is getting out, and more parents, doctors, and nurses are practicing baby massage and reaping its benefits.

By the fifth century B.C., the Greek physician Herodicus was recommending the use of exercise and massage for medical purposes. He was followed in this by his student Hippocrates, later known as the "father" of scientific medicine. Probably the first version of sports massage occurred when Asclepiades, a Greek physician granted Roman citizenship, recommended therapeutic massage and exercises for athletes and gladiators. With its spread from the Greeks to the Romans, massage was transformed into a high art. The Romans created magnificent baths as a centerpiece for massage.

Massage returned to favor in European countries in the sixteenth century when the brilliant French surgeon Ambroise Paré used massage techniques for joint stiffness and the healing of wounds following surgery. Some of the kings of France and England practiced the "Royal Touch," the power to heal disease by touching.

In the early nineteenth century, Pehr Henrik Ling, a Swedish instructor of fencing and gymnastics, developed a theory and technique of soft tissue manipulation, which he called the Swedish Movement Cure, based on the newly discovered knowledge of blood circulation.

Aromatherapy, You, and Your Baby

You wake up on a cool autumn morning in a mountain cabin seeped with the fragrance of sweet pine. You feel refreshed; as you spring out of bed the distinctive aroma of rich coffee arouses your spirit; as you walk through the forest before breakfast the earthy scent of fallen leaves gives you a feeling of comfort and well-being. Aromas around us produce physical and emotional reactions within our bodies, and through aromatherapy—the science of aromas—we have discovered its powerful healing effects. Aromatherapy can be especially therapeutic for you and your baby during pregnancy and after. You can use aromatherapy as a natural way to alleviate certain ailments or the discomforts of pregnancy. For instance, peppermint oil can be used to alleviate morning sickness (peppermint or ginger tea works, too). For sleeplessness, try a blend of lavender, chamomile, and neroli (neroli is an essential oil made from orange flowers). Essential oil drops can be used in a bath, on potpourri, or simply dropped on a cloth to inhale. For massage, dilute essential oils with lotion or a less concentrated oil such as vegetable, sweet almond, or jojoba oil. Try a mixture of sweet almond oil with a few drops of rose oil for a soothing baby massage. Through the sense of smell you can create a stimulating environment for both you and your baby.

The term "massage" itself was introduced in the United States and Western Europe in the late nineteenth century through the work of Dr. Metzger, a Dutchman. His techniques and strokes were accepted by the proponents of the Swedish Movement Cure and became identified with their approach. Today Swedish massage, a system based on Ling's early ideas and many of Metzger's massage strokes or movements, is one of the most common and well-known forms of massage throughout the world.

Similarly, aromatherapy has recently come into vogue, but it has actually been around for centuries in the Middle East, Asia, and India. Aromatic liquid substances, called "essential oils," are extracted from certain species of flowers, grasses, fruits, leaves, and trees. There are about three hundred essential oils, each used for diverse purposes such as medications, cosmetics, flavorings, and fragrance.

> Never use oil on your baby's face, as it can get into her tender eyes, nose, and mouth. Never pour oil directly on your baby's body. Put the oil first on your own hands, and rub your palms together to warm the oil.

Choosing the Best Oils for Baby

Essential oils that have been identified as particularly beneficial or therapeutic for babies include lavender, geranium, chamomile, eucalyptus, and tea tree. These oils have a wondrously calming effect on the nervous system, and babies become more and more content as they savor the loving touch and soothing smell they associate with massage.

Essential oils in their pure state are too concentrated to use directly on the skin, so they are diluted in a base oil. Base oils are vegetable, nut, or seed oils that also have therapeutic qualities. Try to select a baby massage oil that includes natural oils such as soybean, safflower, almond, olive, avocado, grape seed, or sesame.

When using a new oil on your baby or child, test it on a small patch of skin for about thirty minutes to observe whether the area develops a rash, red blotches, or any other adverse reaction. If it does, that oil should not be used on your baby. To remove the oil's residue, clean the area with baby soap and water. Some baby oils and lotions have lots of additives and many contain alcohol, which is not good for a baby's skin (or anyone's, for that matter). So read labels carefully.

Preparing the Scene

Before beginning the Adderly Method of Infant Therapeutic Massage, gather a few things together:

- ❖ massage oil
- ❖ a few extra diapers and towels
- ❖ a change of clothes for your baby
- ❖ a pillow for your baby to lie on
- ❖ a soothing music selection—preferably classical music, (specifically Mozart) which has beneficial IQ effects, which we will discuss later
- ❖ a few small, soft toys for an active baby

Make sure the room you are going to use is heated to about 75 or 80 degrees and is free from drafts. After a massage, it is important to guard against chills, so you might want to wrap your baby in a towel when you're done. Extra diapers are important because many babies urinate during massage, as their sphincter muscles relax.

> In the event that your child needs the comfort of being held before being massaged, by all means do that. In fact, this is a wonderful time to begin a gentle massage of your baby's back, which might make her more amenable to lying down for the massage.

Disconnect the telephone, remove any bulky jewelry that you're wearing on your hands or arms, and make sure your nails are short enough not to scratch your baby. Wash your hands with warm water both for cleanliness and so your touch will be warm and soothing. You might want to take a few minutes to relax yourself by taking some deep breaths, doing some neck rolls, or just closing your eyes. If you're tense, that can be communicated to your baby, even by your touch. This massage really is for both of you, to help you both relax and enjoy a post-massage glow.

Turn the lights down and play your classical tape. Playing the same tape at each massage will teach your child to relax, providing the comfort of routine.

Positioning Your Baby

Positioning your child means putting her in a position that's comfortable for both of you. Tiny babies might even prefer to lie in your lap.

Many parents like to sit on the floor in a modified lotus position, knees bent, soles of the feet together, back supported by furniture.

If this position works for you, pad the area between your legs with thick blankets, making a cradle in which to put your baby. The disadvantage of the modified lotus position is that your baby is not in skin-to-skin contact.

For skin-to-skin contact many parents like to sit with their baby between their outstretched bare legs, the child face up with her feet pointing toward the parent.

Whatever position you adopt, make sure it's comfortable, and adjust it as needed. You don't want to come away from this experience needing a massage yourself!

> Develop your own massage "routine," beginning with the same body part and follow the same sequence to reassure your baby of what is coming.

Massage Basics

All strokes should be long, slow, rhythmic, smooth, and gentle. Where your palms are too large, use your fingertips or thumbs. When we say fingertips, we do not mean the top edges or ends of your fingers; babies sometimes find that touch ticklish, and using the ends of your fingers can also bruise tender flesh. Use the pads of the first joint of your fingers, sometimes referred to as the ball of the finger.

The most important aspect of the Adderly Method of Infant Therapeutic Massage is contact between parent and child. There are no strokes that absolutely must be used—but listen to your child's satisfied coos or watch her facial expression to determine what she prefers. You'll find that your baby responds more to some strokes than others.

Find a sequence of strokes that calm your baby rather than stimulate her. Some people begin at the toes and work up, because their babies find this less threatening, and more instantly soothing.

For the Adderly Method of Infant Therapeutic Massage, we prefer to begin with the head and work down the body, which has the advantage of ensuring early eye contact and of taking the baby's tension down from the head and neck, out through the feet and toes.

> Talking to your baby while you have her heightened attention during a massage contributes to her intellectual development.

Once you're comfortable with your massage technique, feel free to improvise depending on your baby's needs at the time. Legs may be sore after walking, so give them some attention, or if she is recovering from being sick, a back massage might be particularly pleasant.

Be sure to let your baby see your face while you're working. The more eye contact you have with your baby, the better the relationship that develops between you, and the more comfortable your baby will be. The mother who looks at her baby with bright eyes and a smiling face is building her child's self-esteem.

Talk to your baby throughout the massage. A baby will often respond to a parent's voice, touch, and eye contact by producing sounds of her own, looking, moving, or touching.

Tell your baby what you are going to do ("I'm going to massage your feet"), and then what you are doing ("I'm rubbing your toes"). Your calming words will reassure your baby. As she gets older and is able to speak, this time of heightened awareness, when the brain is relaxed yet attentive and receptive to stimuli, is a good time to introduce foreign language words and phrases, starting simply—say, with French words for body parts, or Spanish phrases for your actions. A child's ability to pick up languages is much greater now than it ever will be again, and we'll talk more about increasing this aspect of your child's intellectual potential later in the book.

The Adderly Method of Infant Therapeutic Massage

The Adderly Method of Infant Therapeutic Massage is a guideline, but you will, no doubt, want to extend your repertoire of movements by inventing some of your own or using more strokes in areas your baby particularly enjoys.

The Adderly Method of Infant Therapeutic Massage uses components of Swedish, Indian, and Oriental massage techniques. The Adderly Method seeks a massage synthesis, stimulating and balancing the best techniques of the world. But because the Adderly Method is itself a pinch of this and a pinch of that, feel free to improvise and change the direction of the movements depending on your baby's needs. The rule is simple: the best massage is the massage that works.

If our complete Adderly Method of Infant Therapeutic Massage seems too daunting at first, feel free to make it simpler and shorter, perhaps focusing on a body part a day. Remember, you need only massage your baby for about ten minutes a day to achieve positive effects. In fact, some massage therapists think that more than ten minutes is too much stimulation for a baby, especially newborns. Trust your baby's cues as to whether she needs more or less.

The key to massage is finding the right level of pressure, which for babies needs to be light, and gentle, but firm—what massage therapists call effleurage (eh-FLOO-razh). Let the pressure gently flow from your hands.

Research has shown that preterm infants who received pressure rather than stroking had a greater weight gain. They also showed more relaxation, with a slower heart rate, than babies who received light brush strokes, which raised the heart rate. Many small babies do not enjoy light stroking, possibly because it is experienced as tickling.

During the massage, let your baby be the leader. Never force a massage. Never pry open clenched fists or crossed arms. Massage her elsewhere, help her relax, but follow her lead. Take it slow and easy.

To begin, simply hold the specific body part you want to massage (oil your hands first, if you intend to use oil). Initial holding produces a calming contact and reassurance that your next movements will be all right.

Baby's First Massage

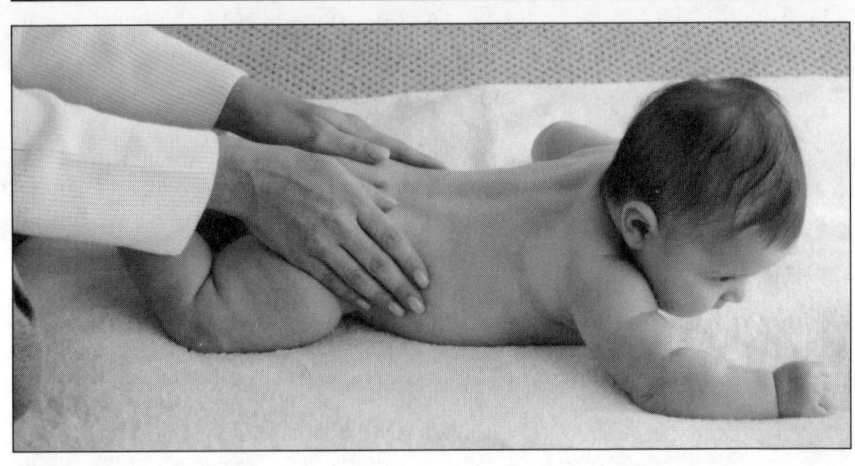

1. *Place your baby face down (on her tummy). Beginning at the shoulder, stroke down your baby's arm, along the side of the torso, over the hip and leg.*

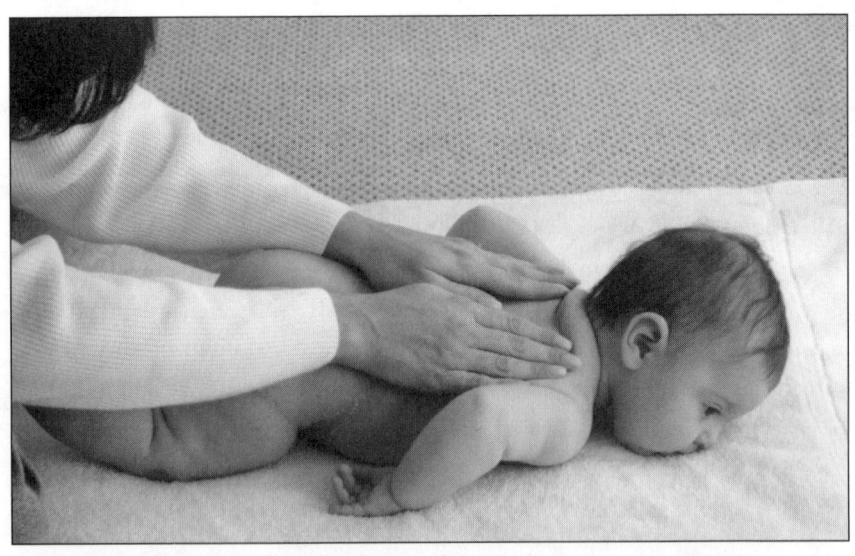

2. *Use a circular stroke on your baby's upper back, moving your hand in a clockwise direction and extending the "clock" down to the center of the back. If you haven't discovered already, this is a very comforting stroke for babies and can relax them even when used through clothes.*

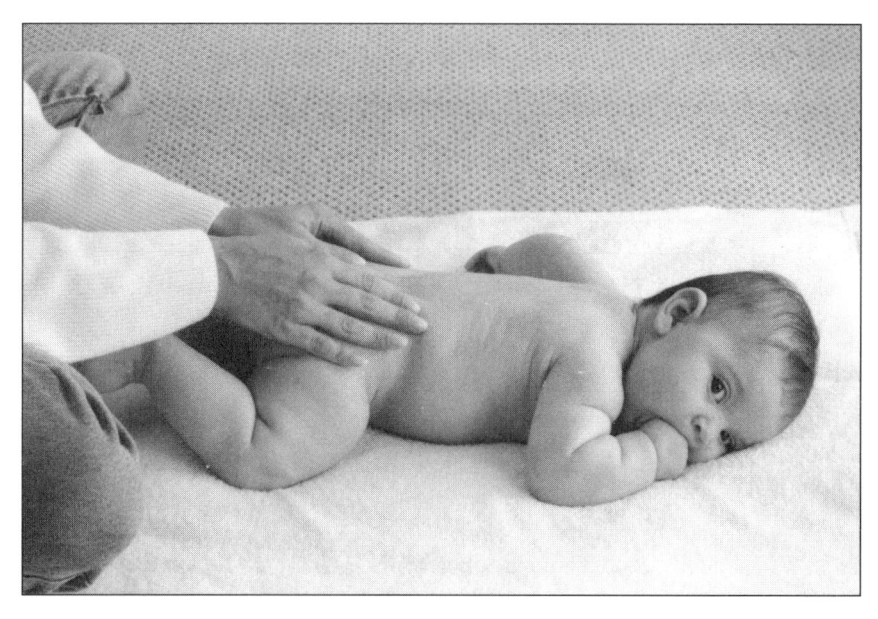

3. *Stroke your baby's lower back at the base of the spine and around the buttocks.*

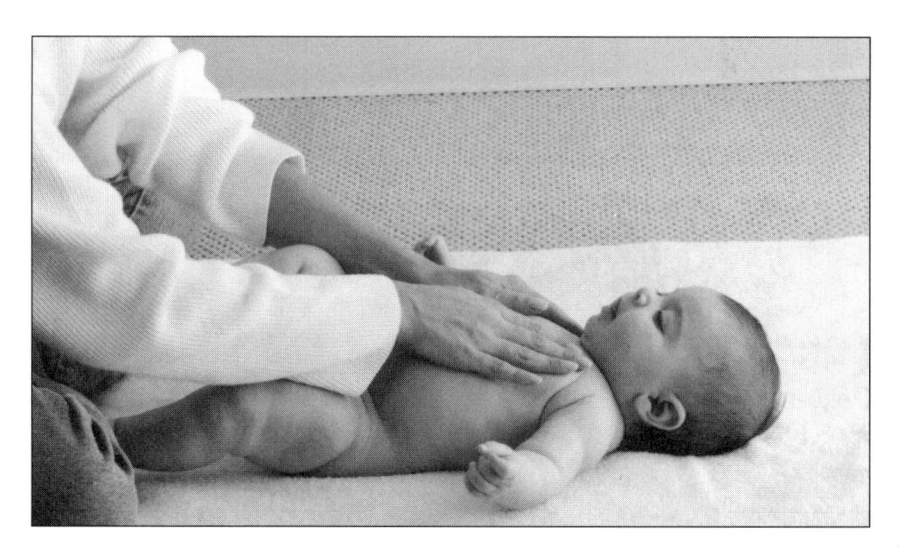

4. *Roll your baby onto her back and stroke gently down the center of the front of the body from the shoulders to the toes. If your baby is not happy to lie on her back at this point, it's all right to roll her over onto the other side and repeat strokes 1 and 2.*

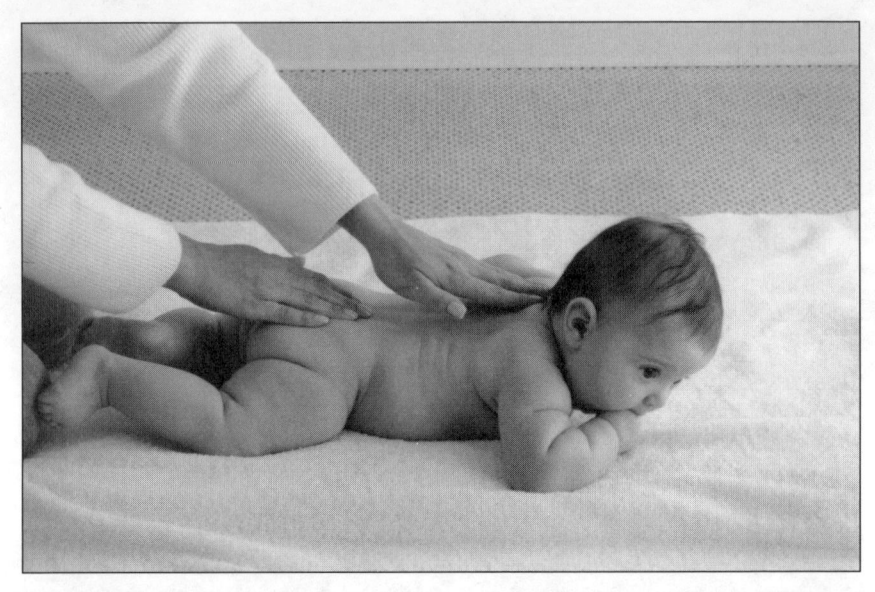

5. *Put your baby on her tummy, or on your tummy so you're lying front-to-front. Stroke straight down the back from the shoulders to the base of the spine. As one hand reaches the spine, begin at the shoulders with the other hand.*

I'm Growing and Ready for More

When your baby is about two months old, has been stroked frequently, and is used to it, both of you might enjoy doing a more extensive massage of all the body parts. Some babies might be ready for this massage earlier.

Repeat each movement in the sequence below at least three times. Observe your baby's body language, and if she does not enjoy the stroke, do not insist on repeating it. Remember, this is supposed to be a relaxing time for both of you.

The Fun Facial

(Do not use oil on the face)

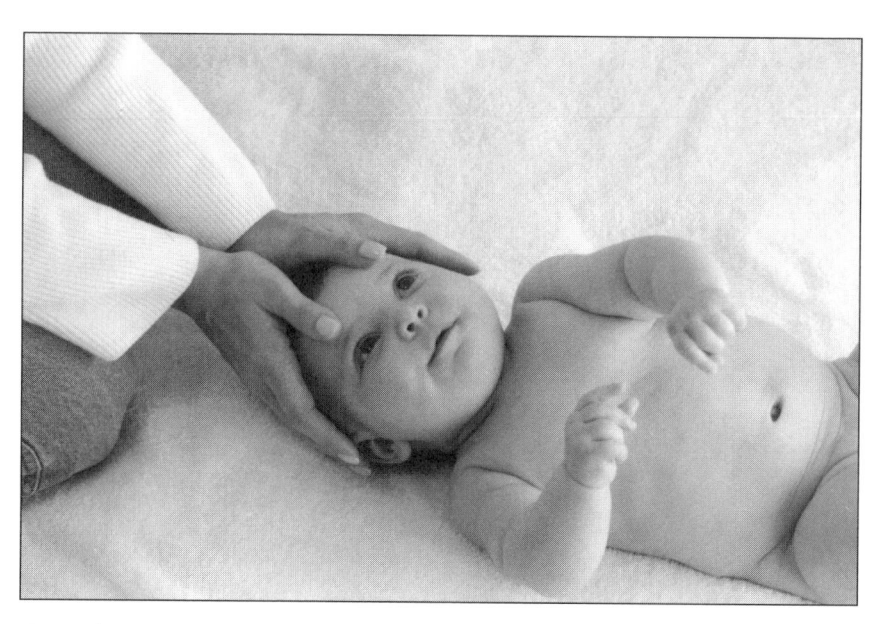

1. *With your baby's head cupped in your hands, use your thumbs to stroke your baby's forehead from the center toward the sides. Keep the rest of your hand relaxed and touching the baby's head.*

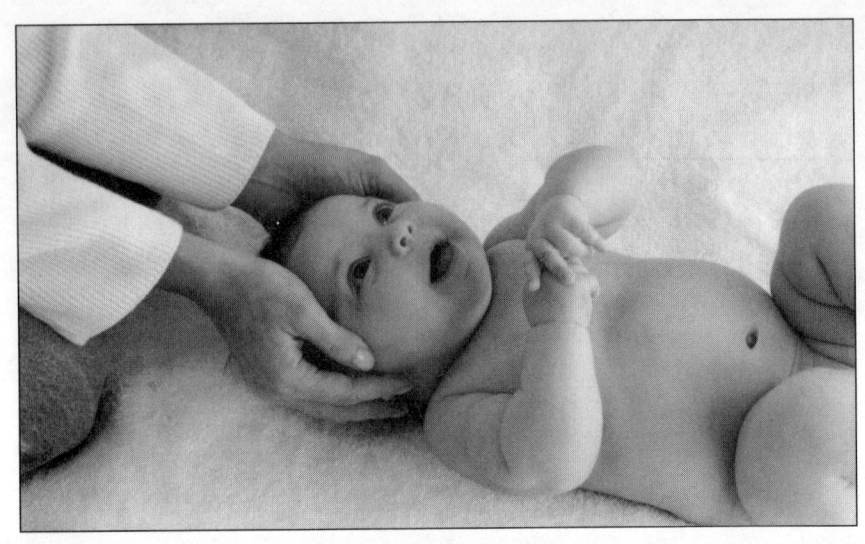

2. *Move down to the cheeks and with your fingers stroke across the cheeks from the nose out and up to the temples. Make light, gentle circles on the temples (counterclockwise for relaxation), then glide your fingers or hands down the sides of the face to the chin.*

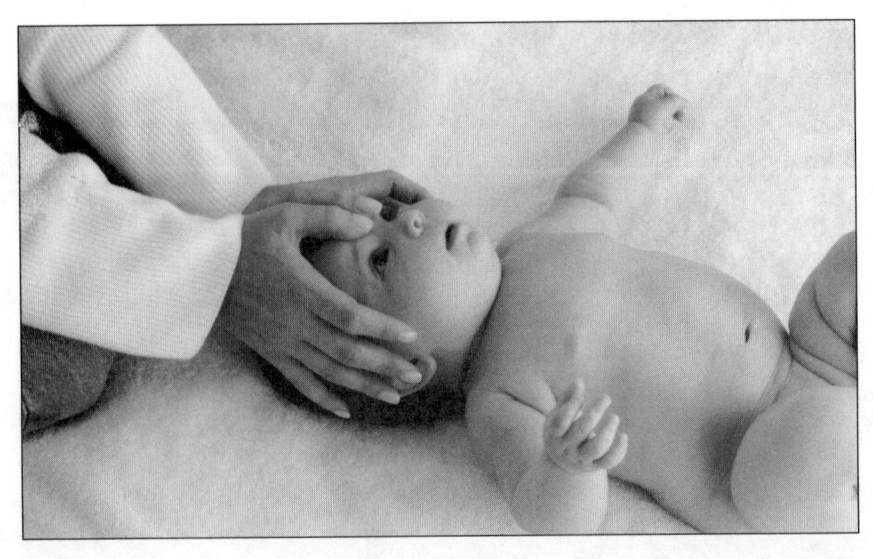

3. *Place your thumbs on either side of the nose. With both thumbs working together, move a short distance upward along the sides of the nose away from the eyes, thumbs coming together over the bridge of the nose and up to the forehead, sweeping your thumbs across the forehead to the temples to finish the stroke.*

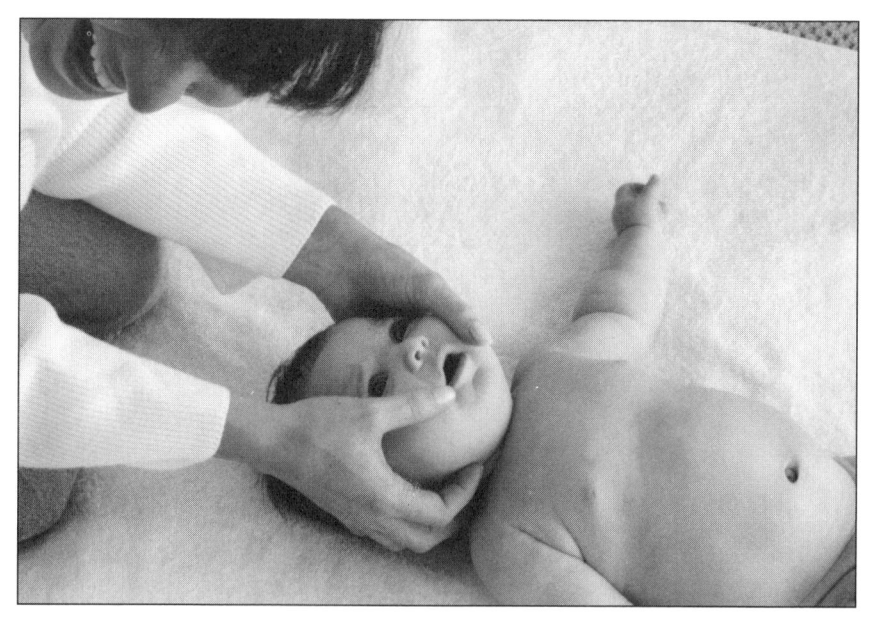

4. *Using your thumbs again, place them above the upper lip, go under the cheek, and stroke up to the ears. If your baby is congested, briefly hold the two points under the nostrils to help relieve congestion before stroking under the cheek and up to the ear.*

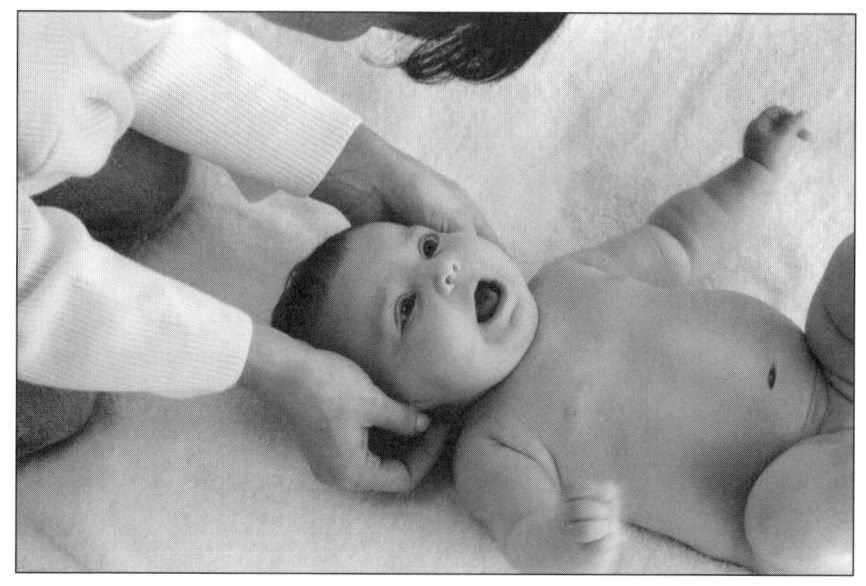

5. *Rub the ears between your fingers.*

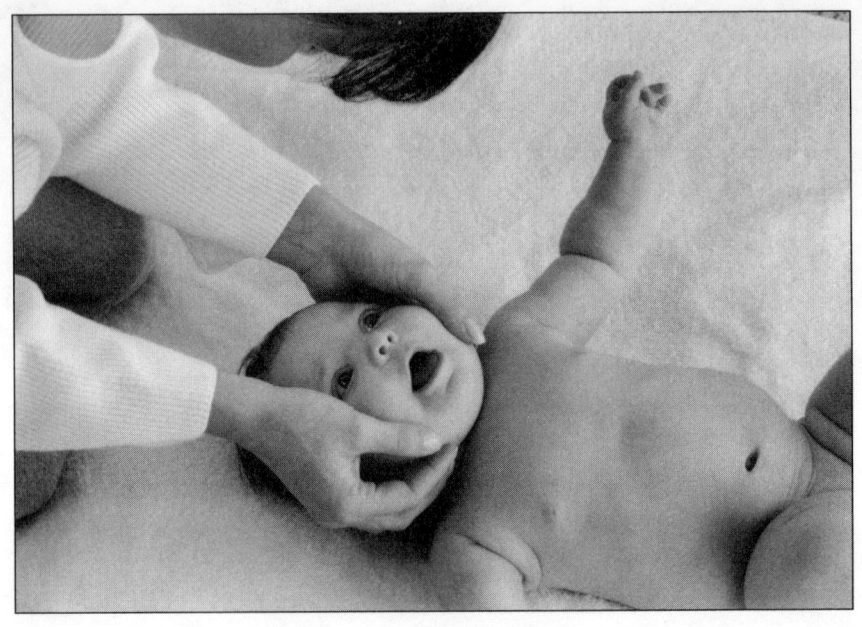

6. *Repeat stroke 4 beginning under the lower lip.*

7. *With one finger, make tiny circles all around the mouth.*

8. *To finish the facial, place your thumbs under your baby's chin and move to the side along the chin. Bring your fingers down and rest your palms on the baby's arms for a few moments.*

> Do not be alarmed if your baby does not at first like the facial massage. Some do immediately, some don't. If your baby doesn't like it, just touch the face gently a couple of times or hold the face with a gentle caress to orient your baby and get her used to facial touching, then move on to other parts of the body.

A gentle brushing across the top of the head and forehead is very soothing for some babies and if you begin it early, may soothe them throughout their childhood. Even if they don't like other parts of their face being touched at first, most babies do enjoy the forehead stroke (stroke 1).

Because the face is always more exposed than the rest of the body, you can do the facial massage anywhere, anytime.

Chummy Chest Work

1. Pour oil on your palms and rub your hands together to warm them and the oil.

2. Place your hands on your baby's upper body to communicate that this is the next place you'll be going to work.

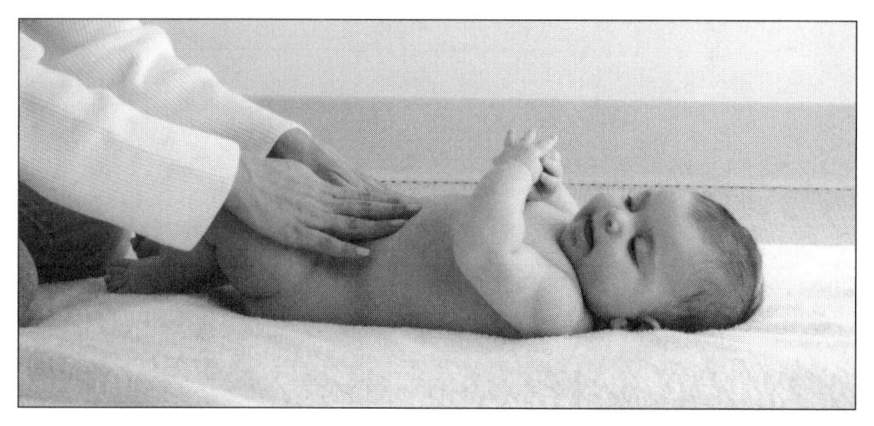

3. With the baby on her back, stroke along the center of the body upward from just above the thighs, over the abdomen, to the shoulders, spreading the oil and massaging at the same time. Glide your hands out to the shoulders, then down the sides of the body to the top of the thighs again.

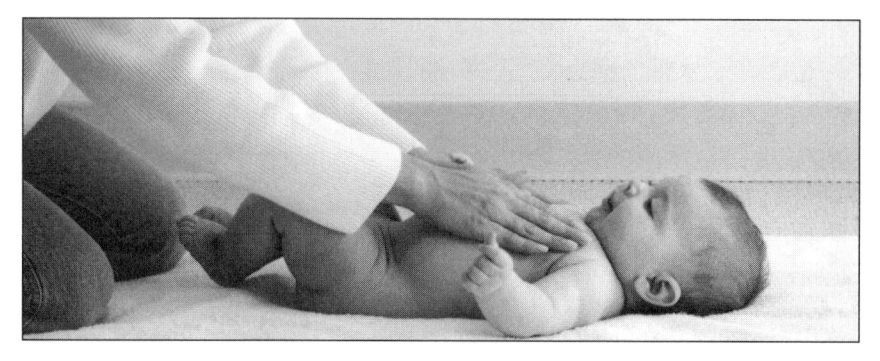

4. With the palm of your hand, make a long sweeping motion down the front of the body from the shoulders to the waist.

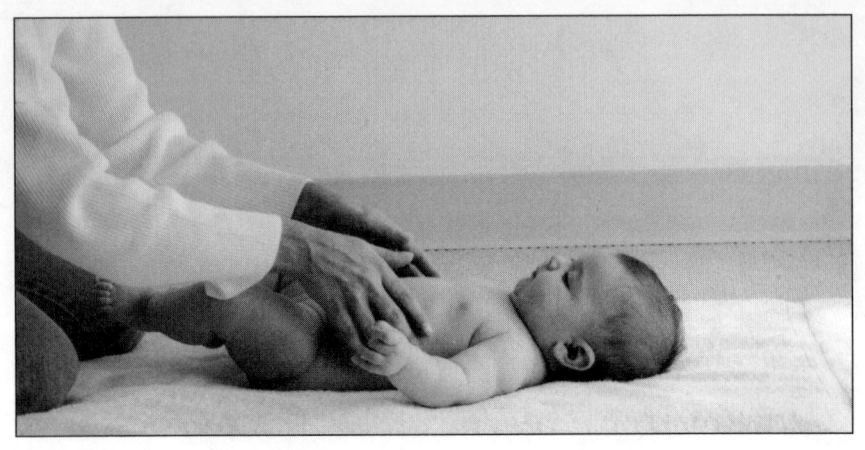

5. *Placing your hands on the center of the upper chest, move them in opposite directions outward toward the sides, stroking down the side of the body and sweeping back onto the chest.*

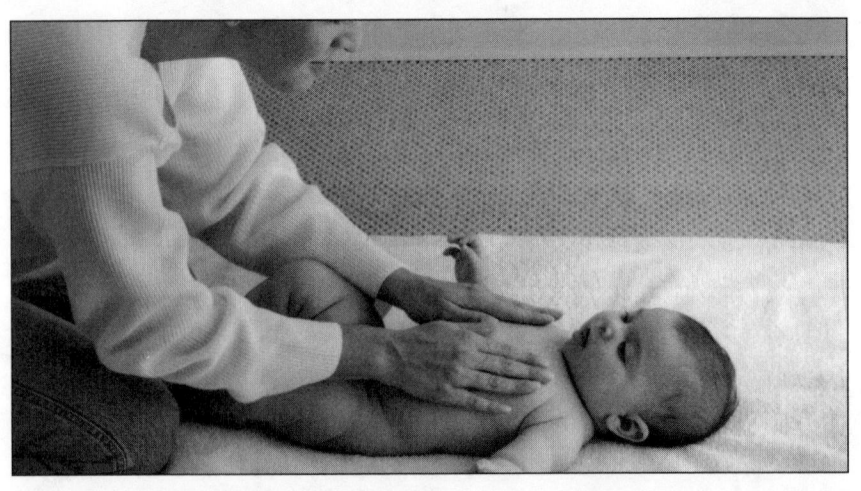

6. *With your fingers flat, create continuous, small spiraling circles over the chest toward the side of the body, then back to the center of the chest. Move down the chest until you have covered all of it.*

Massaging the chest can often help with congestion. It also helps the functioning of the lymph system, which, unlike the heart/circulatory system, does not have a pumping mechanism. Its circulation depends on touch and movement.

Toning the Tummy

(Avoid the navel area until it has healed, simply rubbing around it.)

1. *Pour oil on your palms and rub your hands together to warm them and the oil.*

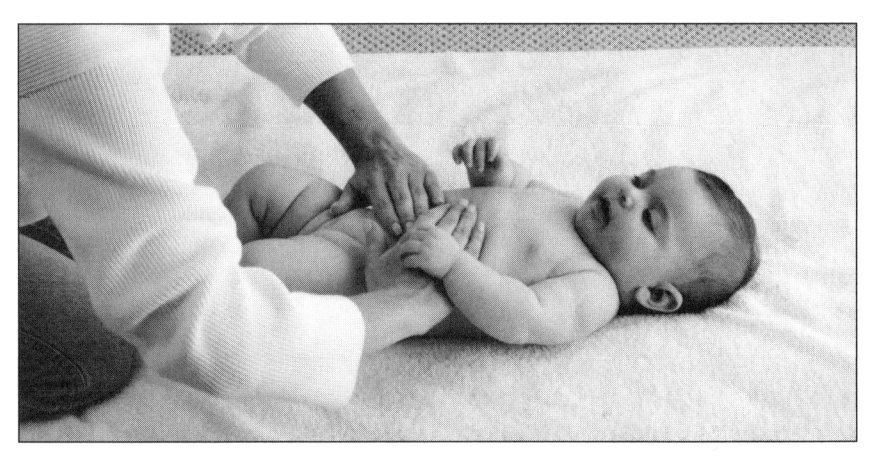

2. *Place your hands on either side of your baby's abdomen (tummy) with your fingers pointing toward each other. Glide the palms of your hands back and forth across the abdomen in a crisscrossing movement.*

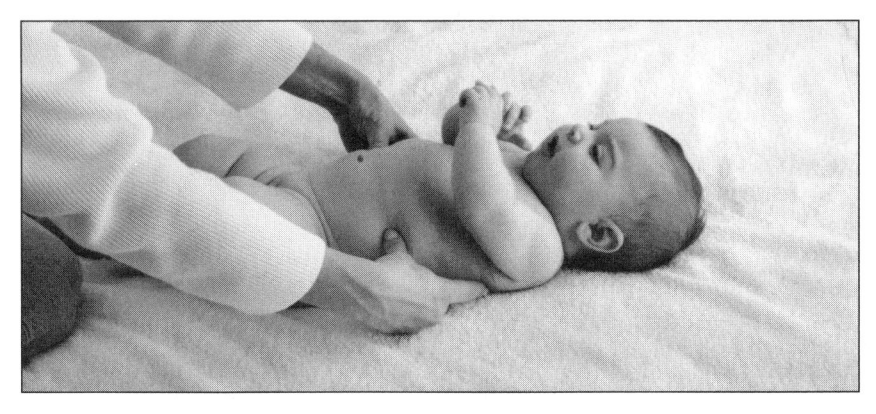

3. *Beginning just below the rib cage, place your thumbs at the baby's center line and stroke to the sides. Continue moving down the abdomen with the same stroke.*

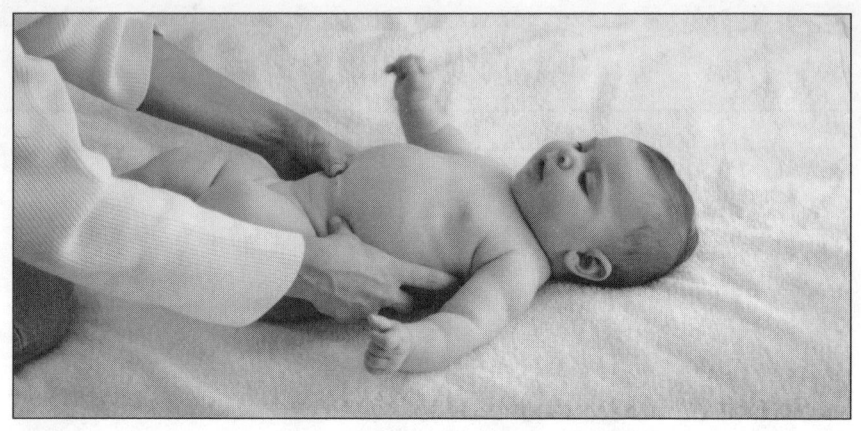

4. *Using both hands, stroke clockwise in a circle around the navel.*

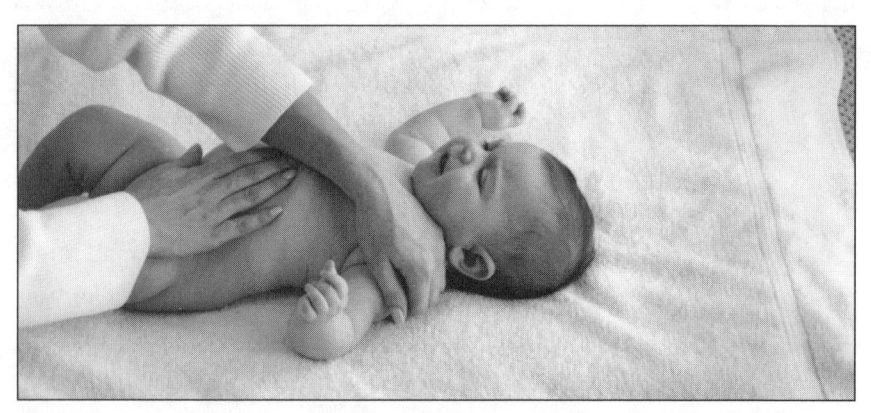

5. *Now move your hands in a double X move. Your right hand starts from the bottom of the trunk and moves diagonally across the abdomen and chest to reach the opposite shoulder. As your right hand reaches the shoulder, your left hand starts its stroke, making the same movement across the length of the torso until it reaches the opposite shoulder. Wait until the left hand has started its stroke before lifting the right hand and placing it at its starting point at the base of the torso.*

Strokes for the stomach generally move clockwise, the same direction that waste moves through the large intestine. Wait at least thirty minutes after a feeding before massaging the stomach and abdomen. Stomach massage relaxes the abdomen, encouraging the elimination of waste and easing gas buildup in a baby's intestines.

Active Arms and Happy Hands

Turn your baby's body so it is perpendicular to you. Arms and hands are another area that many babies do not like at first.

1. *Pour oil on your palms, rub your hands together, and rub the oil along the baby's arm and hand.*

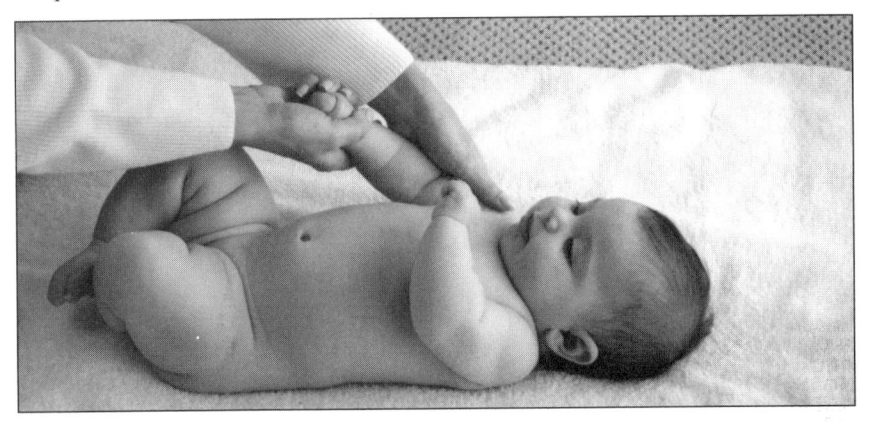

2. *Hold your baby's hand. With your other hand, stroke up the arm from the wrist toward the shoulder.*

3. *Starting at the wrist again with the same hand positions, gently squeeze and release as you move inch by inch from the wrist upward toward the shoulder.*

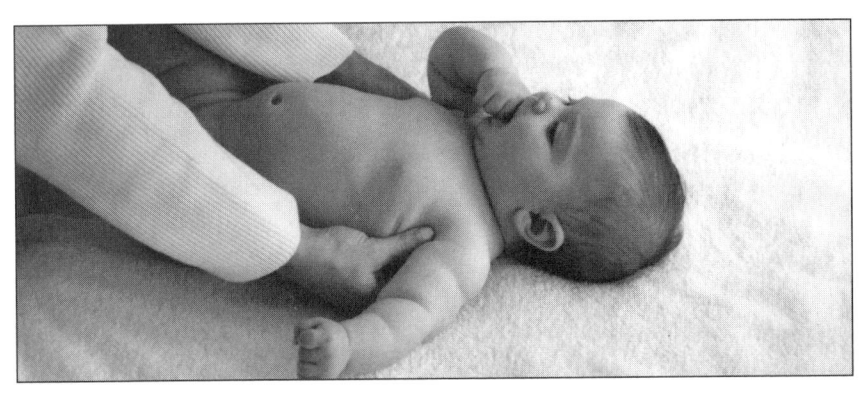

4. *With your fingers, stroke along the connection between the arm and shoulder around and into the armpit. This helps stimulate the lymph system.*

If your baby prefers, an alternative massage is to firmly and evenly work your way down, applying light pressure from the shoulder down to the wrist out through her fingertips.

Working from the shoulder to the hand (away from the heart) is based on the principles of Indian massage. Working from the hand to the shoulder (toward the heart) is the preferred technique in Swedish massage. The Indian method tends to produce more relaxation—the idea is to work tension out of the body, through the extremities, in this case, the fingertips—while Swedish massage is more activating, intended to promote good circulation and body tone.

There's more:

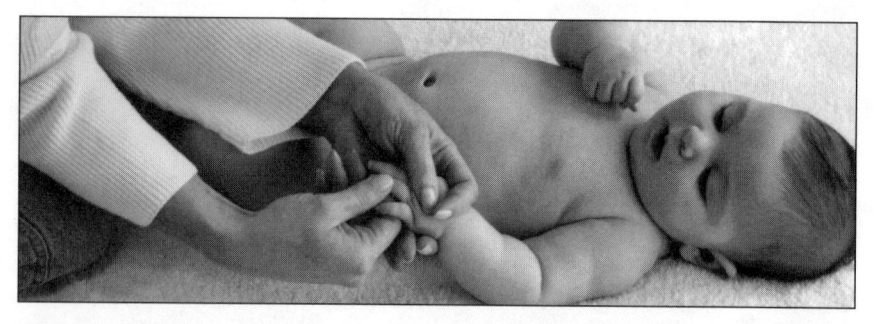

5. *Hold the hand at the wrist and with your other hand slide your thumb (or the palm of your hand depending on the pressure your baby can tolerate) across the back of the hand toward the fingers.*

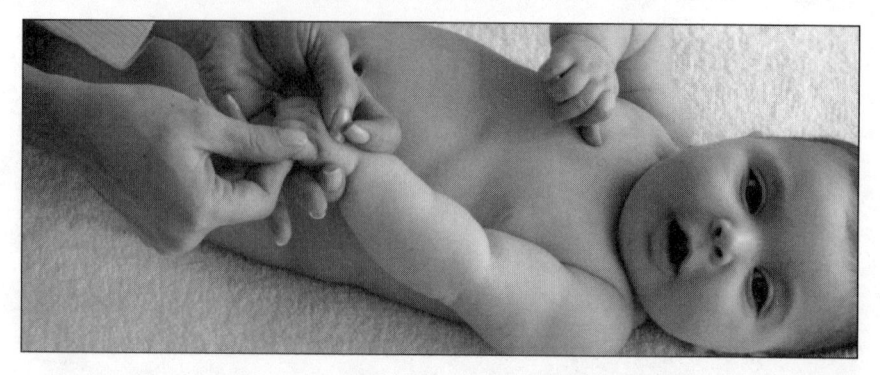

6. *Squeeze each finger on the top and bottom surface between your finger and thumb, and move your fingers toward the end of your baby's fingers, gently squeezing and rotating each of the fingers as you do.*

READY, SET, RUB 43

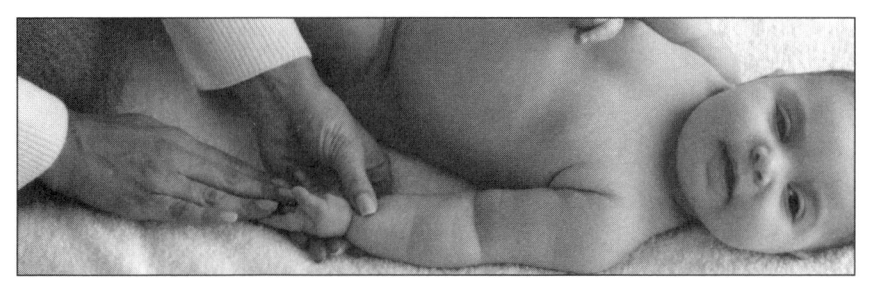

7. *Turn the hand over. Hold at the wrist with one hand and spread your other hand over the baby's palm. Glide your hand downward over the palm and fingers, uncurling the fingers as you slide over them.*

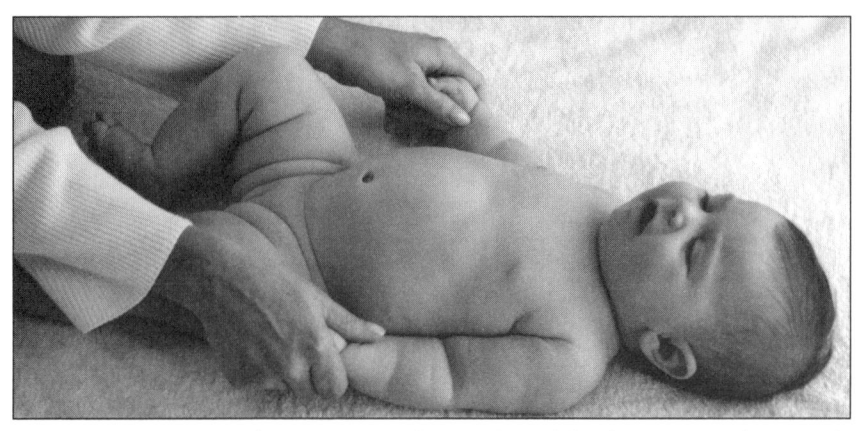

8. *Using your thumbs or your index and middle fingers, simultaneously make small circles around the wrist bones and into the palm of the hand.*

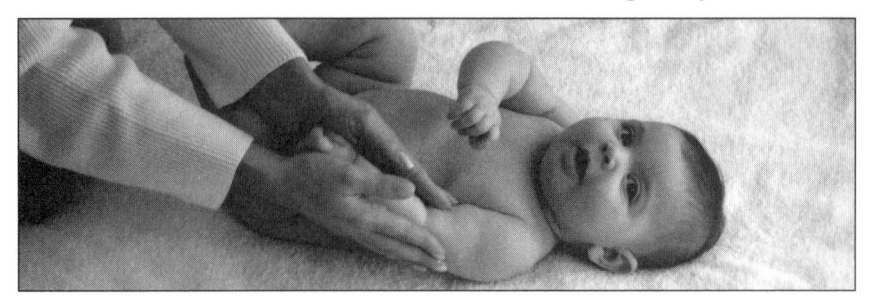

9. *Moving from upper arm to wrist, cup your hands and roll the arm you are finishing back and forth between your hands. Pause for a moment, then repeat the movement. Maintain one hand at the wrist while you move the other hand to the upper arm. This ensures continued contact and is reassuring to the baby.*

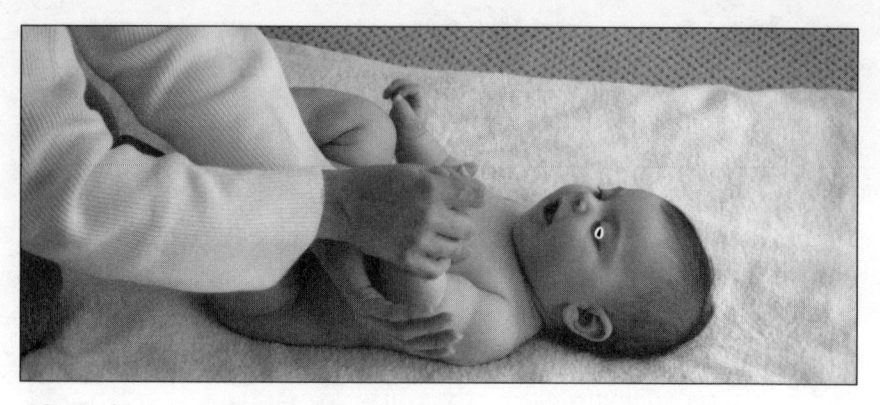

10. *Hold the arm at the elbow and hand, bounce it gently, asking your baby to relax the arm. Say, "relax" and as soon as you feel a relaxation in the arm, praise your baby. "Great, you relaxed your arm." This helps the baby to further associate your touch with relaxation.*

11. *Turn your baby around so the other arm is near you and repeat strokes 1-10 for the second arm.*

Hands are your baby's most important tool for active exploration of the world. Stroke 6 is a beginning step in helping your child identify his separate fingers, and stroke 7 helps your baby open her fist in readiness for grasping objects with an open hand. It is especially useful in the first month after birth.

READY, SET, RUB 45

Lovely Legs and Fabulous Feet

1. *Pour oil on your palms, rub your hands together, and rub the oil along the baby's legs and feet.*

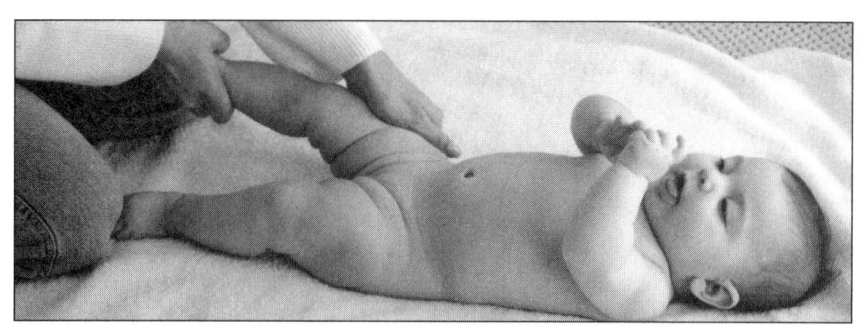

2. *Hold your baby's foot/leg in one hand and beginning at the ankle, stroke up the outside of the leg to the torso (stroke toward the heart).*

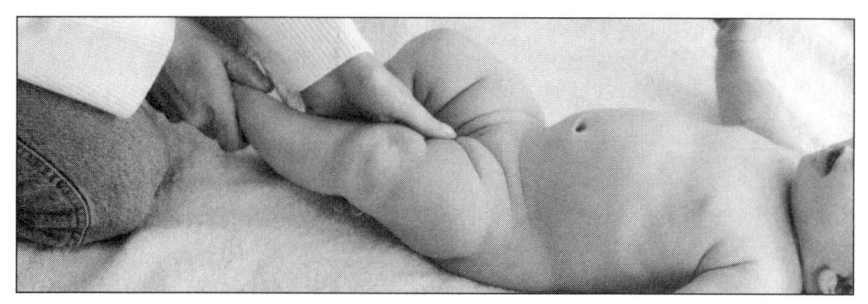

3. *Change hands and, beginning at the ankle, stroke up the inner leg to the torso (stroke toward the heart).*

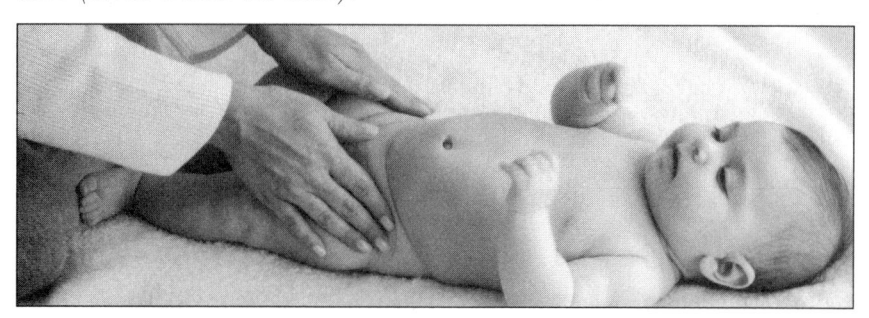

4. *Stroke along the groin line between the torso and the thigh to help the flow of the lymph system.*

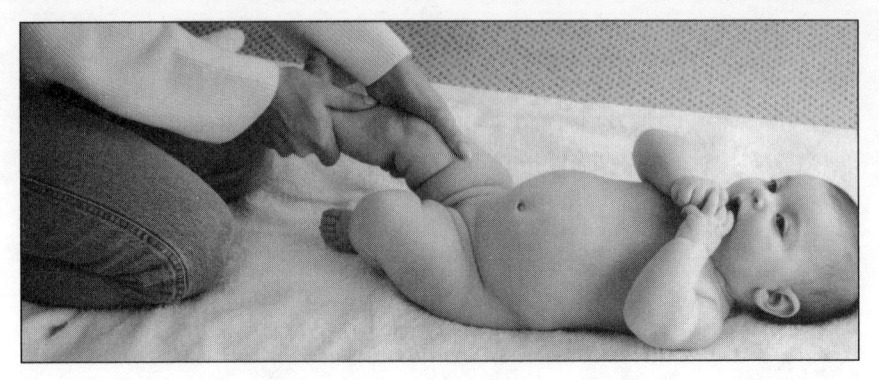

5. *With both hands, gently squeeze and release the leg, moving hand over hand from torso to foot.*

As with the arms (See stroke 2 of Active Arms and Happy Hands), if your baby prefers, an alternative way is to pull firmly and evenly down the leg and out through the toes. Work from torso to foot to relax your baby, or from foot to torso to give her the glow of well-being that comes from stimulated blood circulation.

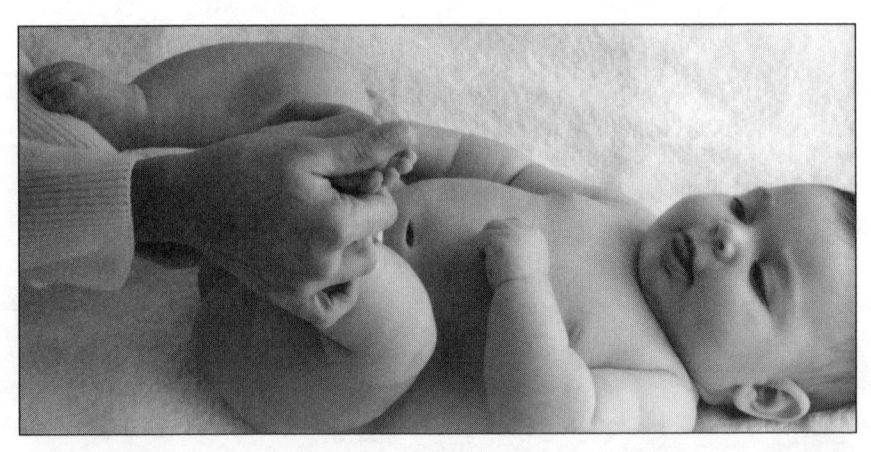

6. *Stretch the leg up. Hold the ankle with one hand and glide your hand over the sole of the foot from heel to toe. Squeeze each toe between your finger and thumb and gently roll or rotate it. It's likely that for the newborn you will cover the entire toe, but as your baby grows, extend this movement all the way to the end of your baby's toes. Also, as your baby grows older you might want to use your thumb to push on the sole of the foot.*

READY, SET, RUB 47

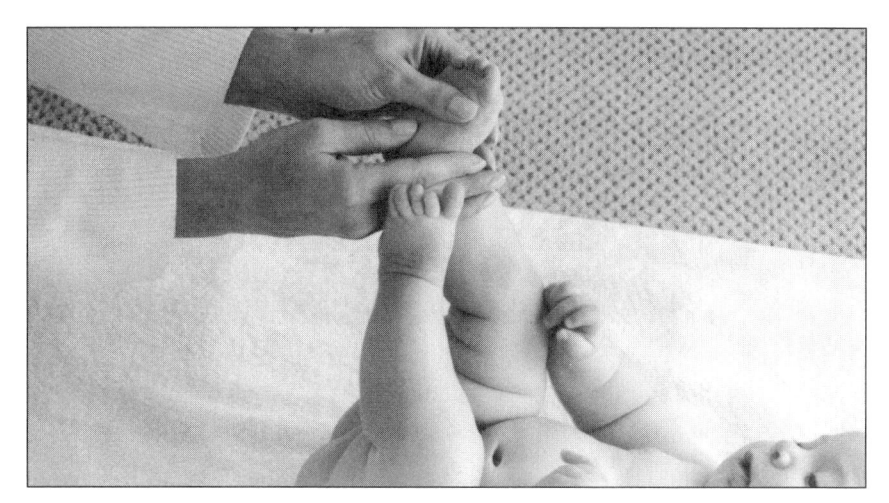

7. *Using one finger, or your thumb, make tiny circles in the center part of the heel.*

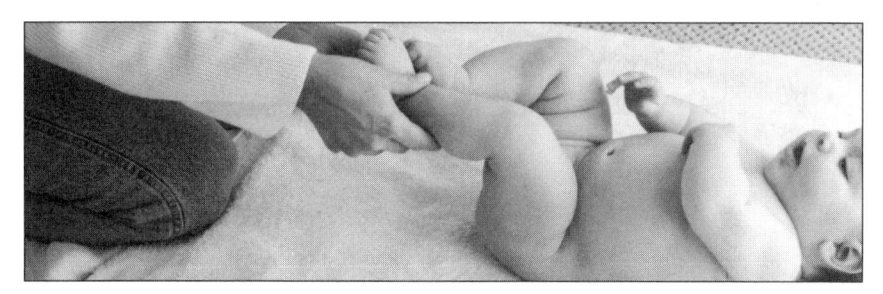

8. *Hold the foot in both hands and make small circles all around the ankle with your thumbs.*

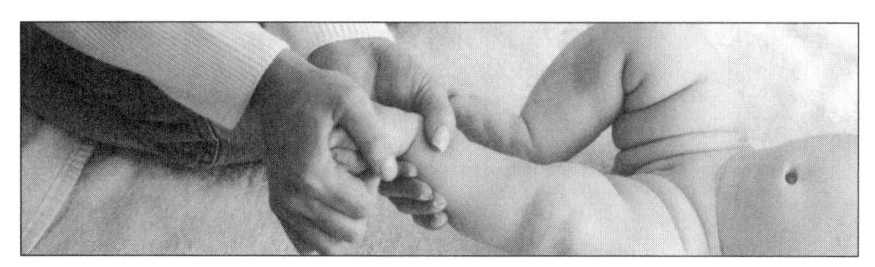

9. *Holding the foot in one hand by cupping it around the heel, push along the top of the foot toward the ankle. Depending on the age and comfort of the child, use your thumbs or the palm of your hand.*

10. *Turn the ankle in circles clockwise then counterclockwise to keep the ankle joint flexible.*

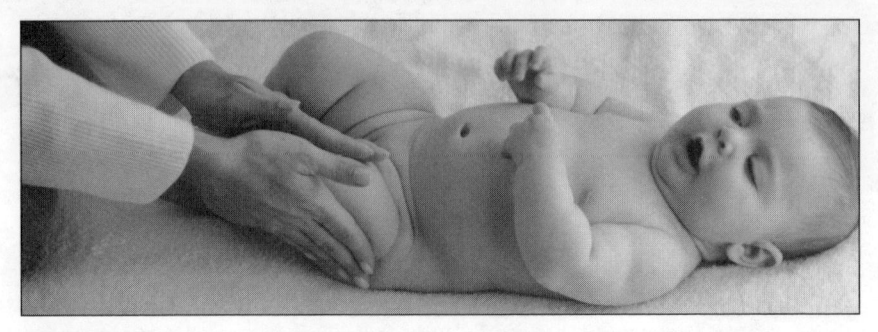

11. *Cup your hands and roll the leg you are finishing between your hands from thigh to ankle. You and your baby may also enjoy shaking the leg a little as you do this. Pause for a moment, then repeat the movement. As with the arm, maintain one hand at the ankle while you move the other hand to the thigh to ensure reassuring contact.*

12. *Hold the leg at the ankle and knee and bounce it up and down gently. Ask your baby, as you did with the arms, to let go and relax, and be sure to praise her when she does.*

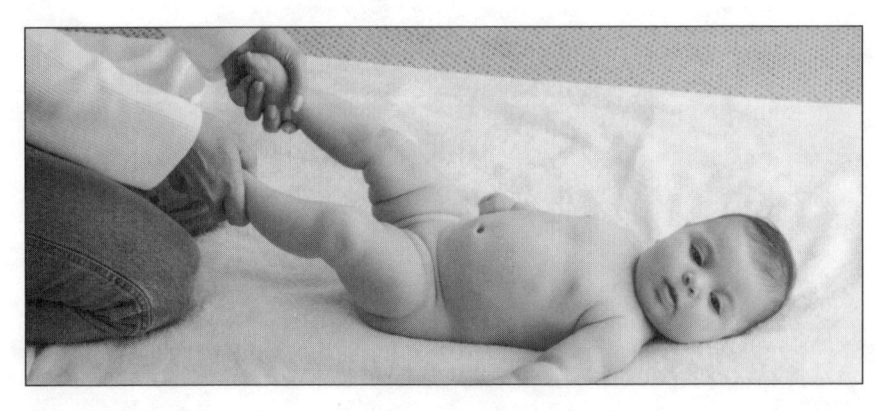

13. *Repeat steps 1 through 12 on the other leg.*

14. *Straighten both legs out and give them a little shake.*

If your baby does not enjoy the stimulation caused by the moving pressure on the sole of the foot in stroke 6, simply use your palm to apply a steady pressure to the bottom of the foot. Stroke 4 is also a natural time to play toe games such as "This Little Piggy."

A Beautiful Back

1. *Turn your baby on her tummy. She can be straddled across your lap or a padded floor—whatever is more comfortable for both of you.*

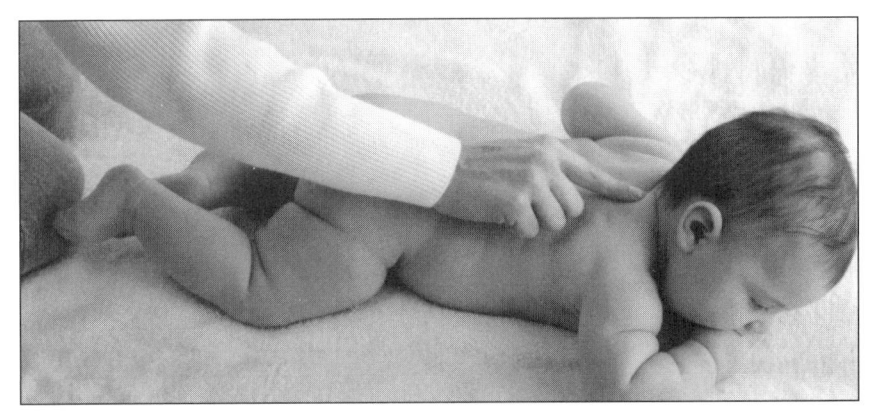

2. *Using one fingertip, make small circles all along the occipital crest at the base of the head.*

3. *Rub a little oil onto your hands and then onto the back and buttocks, starting at the shoulders and continuing down to the buttocks.*

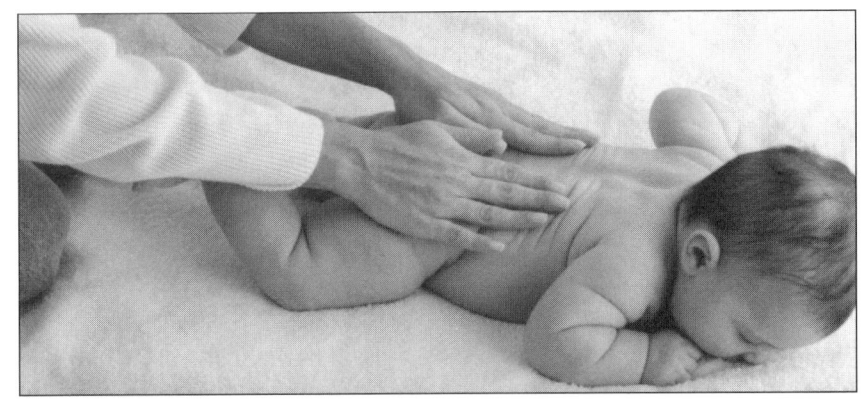

4. *Starting at the feet, glide both hands up the back of the legs, over the bottom, and up the back.*

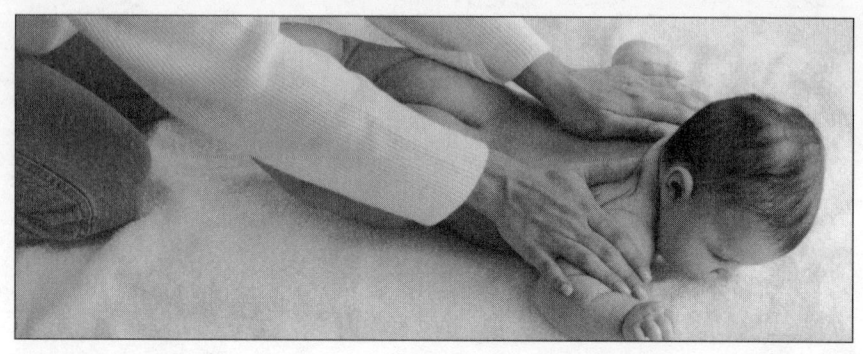

5. Glide your hands out across the shoulders, down the arms and down the sides of the body.

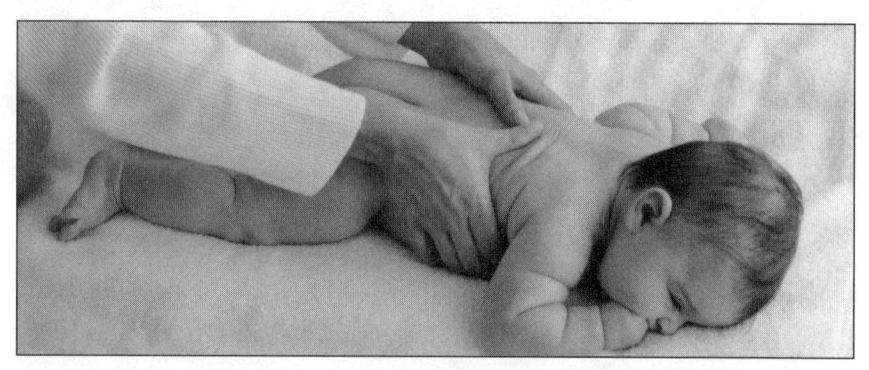

6. With your thumbs on either side of the spine (not on the spine), glide them up your baby's back along the little "valleys" or indentations on either side of the spine.

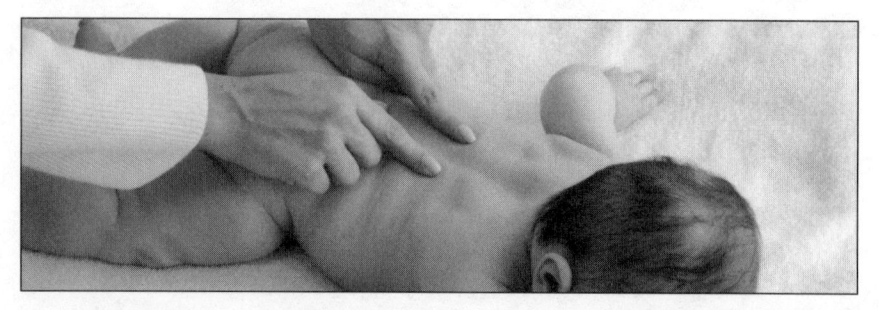

7. An alternative movement to 6 above, is to place the fingertips of the forefinger of each hand on either side of the spine and make three little jiggles up and down. Slide the hand down slightly and make three more jiggles. Continue until you have covered the entire back to the base of the spine

8. *Using a crisscrossing movement, glide your hands back and forth across the back and buttocks, moving from shoulders to bottom and then down.*

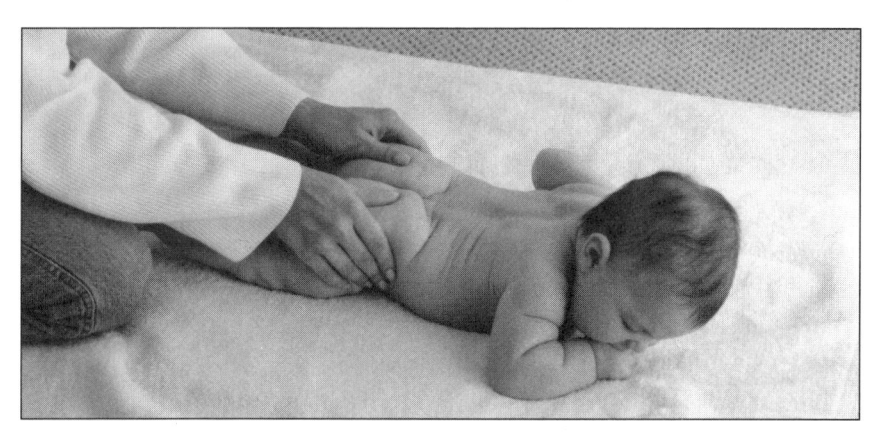

9. *Glide your hands around each buttock, kneading it gently with thumb and fingers (babies use their buttocks a lot in their movements). Then using both hands, rhythmically pat your baby's bottom.*

10. *Holding your baby's bottom in one hand, "swoop" down the back with the other hand.*

11. *Using strokes more light than any of the preceding, glide your hands softly and smoothly down your baby's back, one hand following the other, down the legs, then back to the neck.*

Baby "Aerobics"

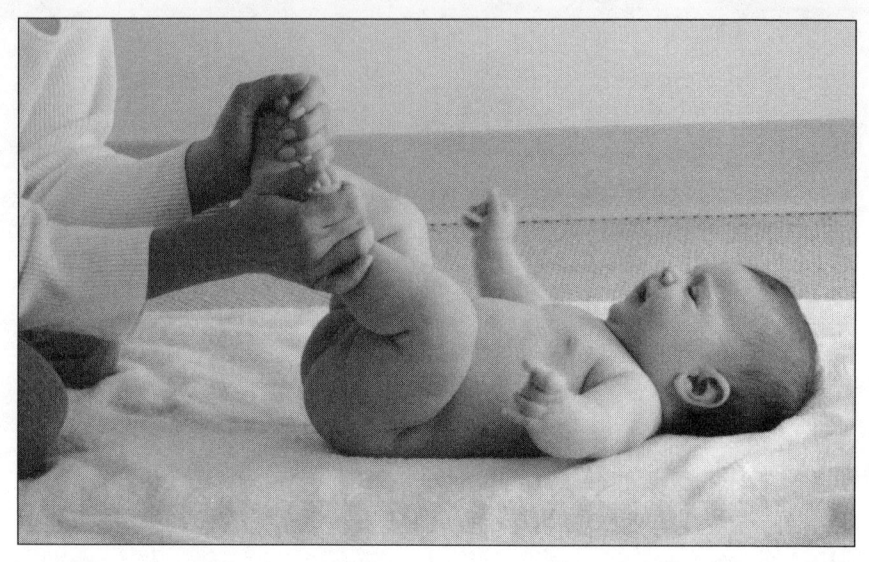

1. *Hold your baby's feet in each of your hands and bend and stretch each leg. Discover how fast or slow your baby prefers to have this movement done.*

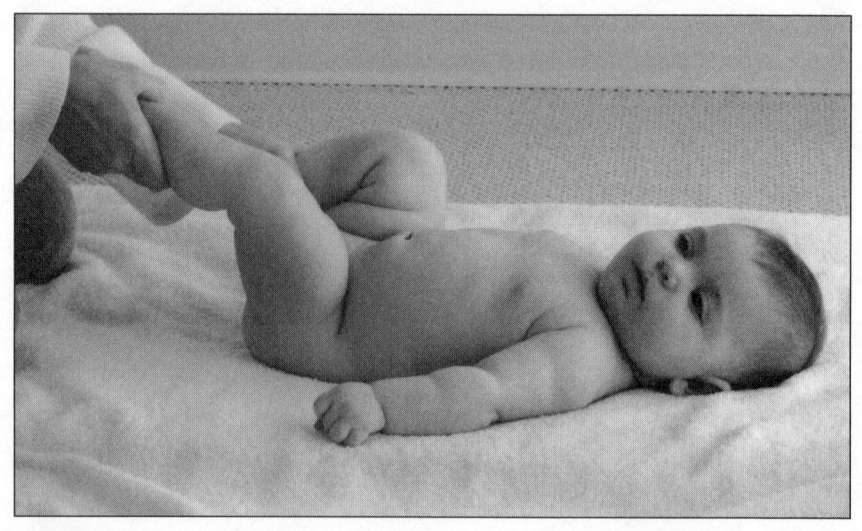

2. *Push the legs up to the belly, bending them as you go and then straighten them out again.*

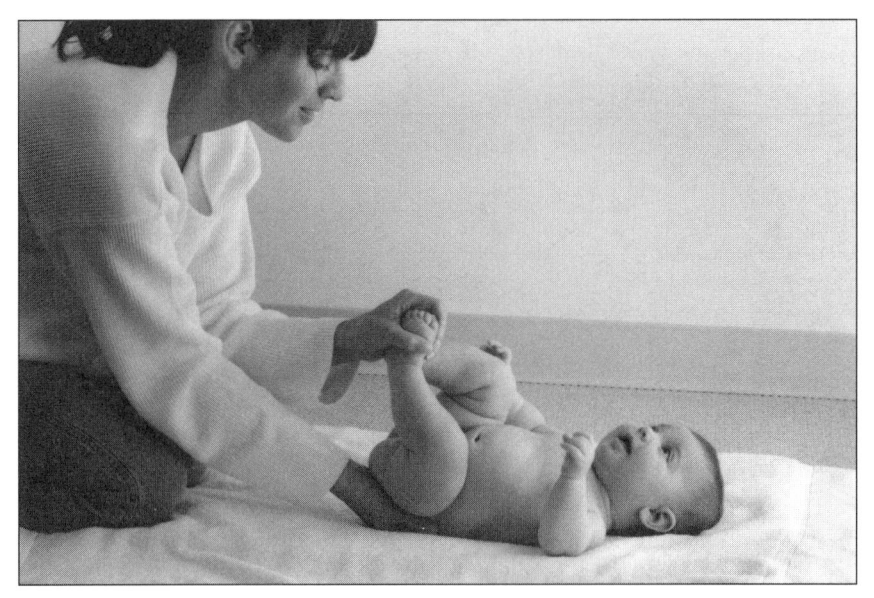

3. *Clasp the soles of your baby's feet together, letting the knees bend outward and rocking your baby from side to side to loosen the hip joints. After a few moments of this, continue the rocking motion with one hand and with the palm of the other hand massage around the base of the spine.*

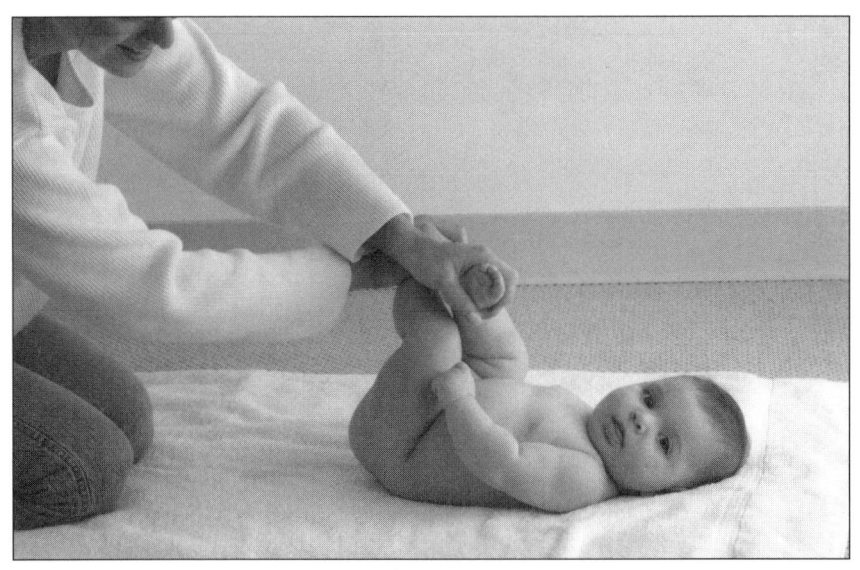

4. *Bend one leg and move it toward the knee of the other leg. Repeat with opposite leg.*

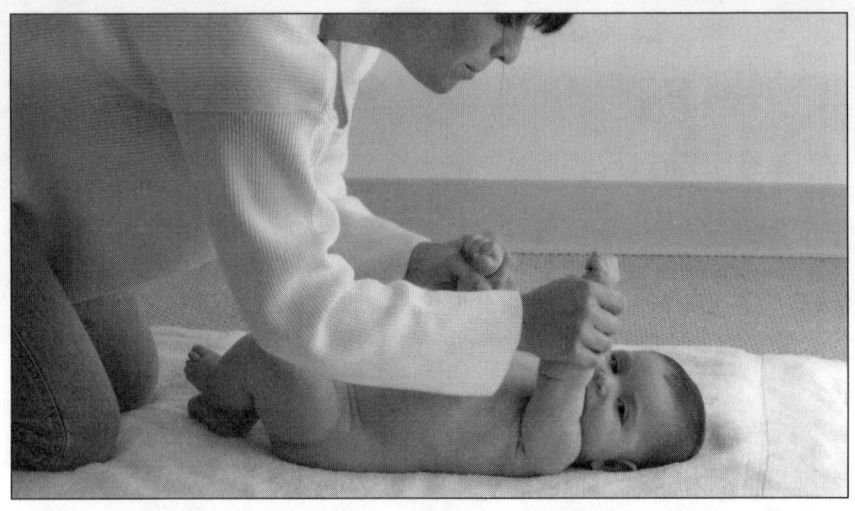

5. *Holding an arm in each hand, move them simultaneously up and down (stimulates the lymph system).*

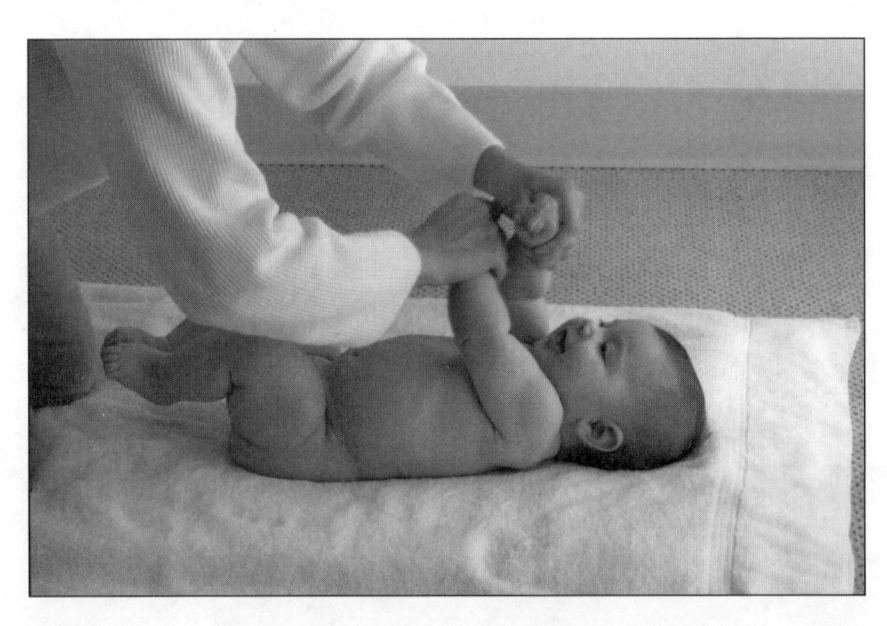

6. *Holding your baby's arm in each of your hands, move the arms straight out to the side, stretching gently. Then bring them in toward the chest and cross them over one another at the center of the body (stretches the upper back and spine). Alternate which arm is on top and which on bottom.*

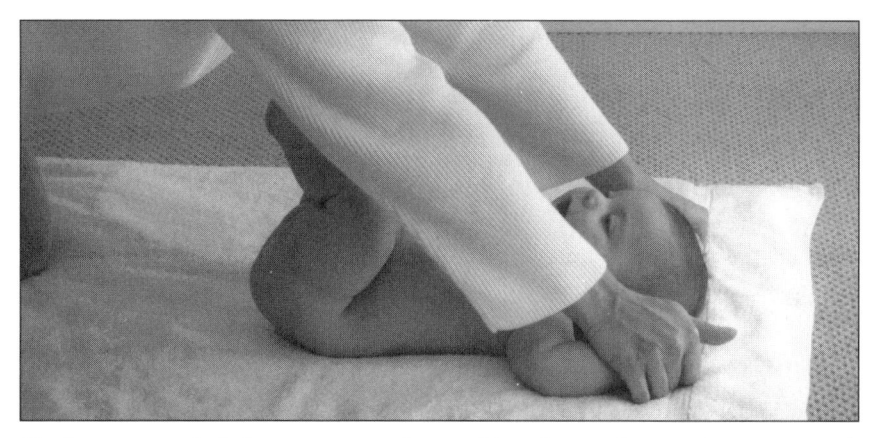

7. *Bring your baby's arms up in front of her face and cross them over each other, alternating which arm is on top. Raise her arms up above her head and stretch them gently, then lower.*

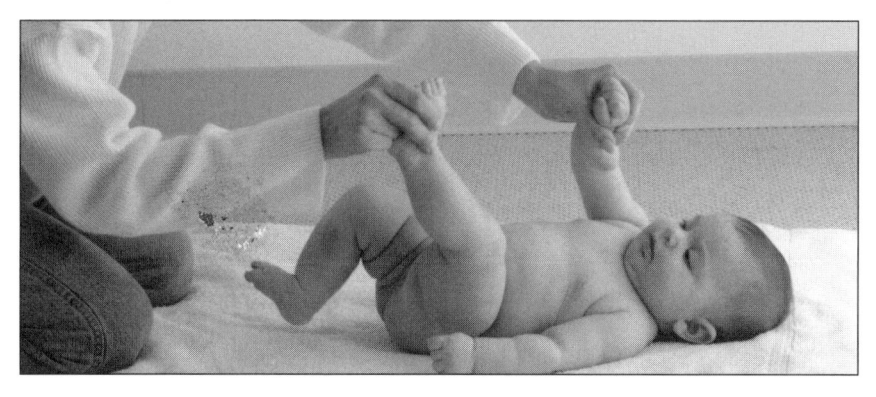

8. *Holding the opposite arm and leg bring them together over the torso, then open back to original position. Repeat three times.*

Babies love these gentle passive movements, which extend and relax the muscles. There is no particular order in which to do them, and one or more of them can be done at any time with your baby dressed or not. The movements also help strengthen and relax your baby's back muscles. Movements 3 and 4 are great for keeping the hip joints flexible. The arm/leg touching in 8 is especially good to loosen the back if your baby has been in a baby carrier or car seat.

When your child is fully mobile and makes his own opportunities to stretch and exercise, you can omit these movements.

As Baby Grows, Change the Massage to Meet Her Needs

During the first three months after birth, babies tend to keep their arms and legs close to their body and may not like the opening movements that extend their arms away from the body or stretch their legs. Gradually, however, as they become more comfortable with the world and with their bodies, they will open up more and be more comfortable having you stretch out their arms and legs.

At three months, facial massage is particularly helpful for a baby that has gathered stress there through crying, teething, and sucking. It's at this stage that you might also be confronted with active, kicking legs, and swinging arms.

Sometimes during the sixth to twelfth month, your baby might decide she does not like being on her back for the massage. She might want to sit up. Now that you've gained skill in your massage techniques, this is the time to improvise and massage as much or as little as your baby will allow, or change your strokes or sequence to adapt to your baby's expanding mobility. Don't become frustrated, and by all means continue your practice of daily massage. As your baby begins to stand upright and walk, massage will be even more beneficial for maintaining flexibility and removing tension.

> **Never too Late**
> If your baby is not a newborn, you can still begin massage now. One of the values of massage is that people of all ages can enjoy and benefit from it. It's never too late to start.

By the time your baby is two years old, she might be ready to direct your massage, informing you of her likes and dislikes.

You'll be relieved to know that after the wiggles and demands of the two-year old, if you have persevered, your three-year-old is more likely to lie still and allow you to give her a complete massage. Modesty begins around this age, and your baby might be more comfortable wearing underwear during the massage.

Special Strokes for Special Needs

The Fussy Baby

This technique is good if your baby gets fussy during a massage, or if there is a particular time of the day your baby gets fussy.

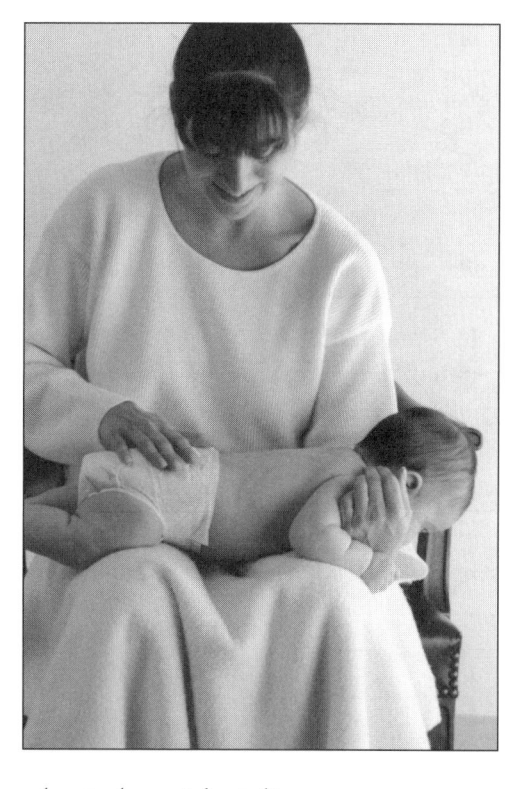

1. *Put the baby across your lap, supporting the head with your arm under the chin and around the sides of the baby, so she can rest her head on your arm and look ahead or close her eyes.*

2. *In this position, rock the baby gently and/or pat the back and buttocks rhythmically.*

3. *An alternate position is to put the baby on her back, and holding her feet, rock her body back and forth, left to right.*

The Baby with Colic

If your baby has colic, some of the massage strokes and movements below might help relieve the gas and discomfort. It is especially good to use an hour before bedtime or when your baby usually gets fussy.

If your baby has gas or a tight belly, this massage may hurt a little, so don't be surprised if your baby cries. *However, if your baby registers a strong, continuous disapproval, don't continue.* Massage your baby twice a day for at least two weeks to determine if this massage helps. Use each stroke six times unless otherwise indicated by your pediatricion. All sweeping movements should be from the rib cage down, and all circular movements should be in a clockwise direction since that is the direction of digestion.

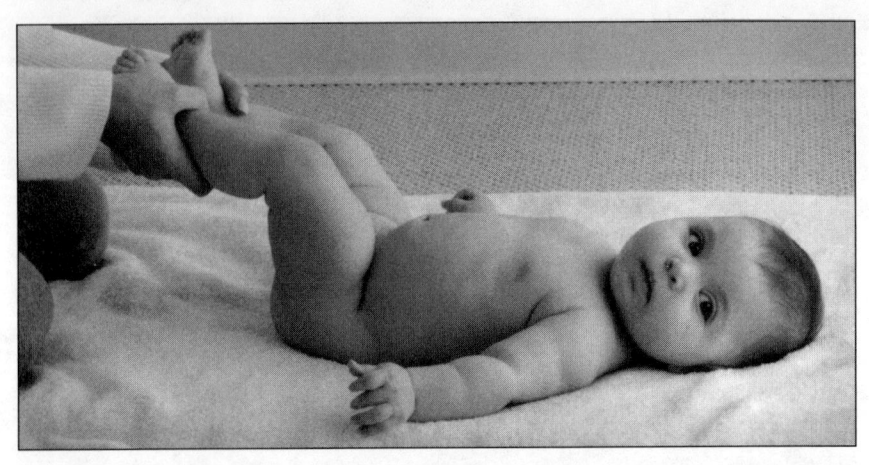

1. *The most simple technique is to hold the legs so the baby's knees are together, and bend the baby's legs up toward the chest, hold a few moments, and then bring them down again, straightening the legs out. Do this about three times.*

2. *With the tips of your fingers, make small circles on the abdomen, moving clockwise around the tummy. If there is a spot that feels firmer or more dense than others, give it a little extra care.*

3. *Repeat step 1 once.*

4. *With the fingertips, make small circular strokes below the rib cage.*

5. *Repeat step 1 once.*

6. *Using the palms of your hands, and alternating hands, "scoop" or stroke down from the stomach toward the feet and repeat.*

7. *Repeat step 1 once.*

8. *Left of the navel and diagonally down toward the left just above the groin is the ileocecal valve, the entry to the last part of the small intestine. It can sometimes get blocked, so use those little circular strokes to keep it open.*

> Colic can be a sign of a more serious condition, so be sure to consult your doctor.

Sometimes holding your baby in what massage therapists call the "football hold" will help relieve some of the pressure. You hold your baby like a football, supporting the head and back with one arm. Place the other hand over the abdomen. Gravity, body weight, and your hand(s) put slight pressure on the abdominal area. It also may help to rock your baby while holding him this way.

The Congested Baby

This is a technique that physical therapists sometimes use for a baby with congestion.

1. *With your baby sitting upright in your lap and supported with one hand, cup your other hand and pat the baby's back for about a minute. Massage therapists call this tapotement or percussion.*

2. *Now pat the baby's chest with your cupped hand.*

3. *Lean your baby forward at a 45-degree angle. Cup under one armpit. Release, and then cup under the other armpit, and release. Then pat the back in this position.*

Do not be alarmed if your baby coughs or spits up phlegm. This is exactly what you want to happen.

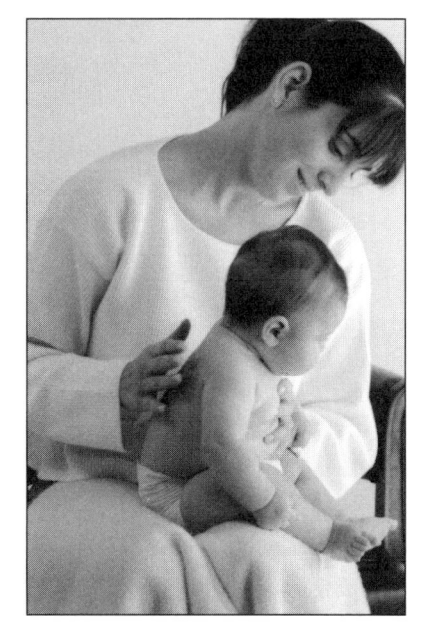

It might be useful now if we turn to the testimonials of parents who have seen the benefits of Infant Therapeutic Massage.

CHAPTER 4

The Experience of Parents

Here are the experiences of some parents whose children have benefitted from baby massage. Their experiences might mirror your own.

Zoe

Zoe is the nine-month-old daughter of an insurance salesman, Michael, and of Lucy, a primary school teacher. Zoe's mother took a three-month maternity leave after her baby was born.

Lucy started massaging Zoe when she was about two weeks old.

"There were parts of it Zoe liked right away," Lucy says, "even though I was kind of nervous, but she didn't really seem to like having her face touched. So I just sort of made light circles on her forehead and the top of her head. That seemed to work okay."

After the massage Lucy gave Zoe her bath, and Zoe was almost falling asleep before they got finished. "She was so relaxed at the end of the massage, that I probably shouldn't have tried to give her a bath at that time," says Lucy. "I, on the other hand, was a nervous wreck trying to figure out how to do the massage and if I was doing it right."

Zoe slept a little longer than usual that day, so Lucy decided to try again the next day. "This time it was almost like she knew what was going to happen. She cooed, but, of course, she did that most of the time when you looked at her," says Lucy. "I think the main difference was that I had resolved not to work so hard and to just do what seemed to be satisfying for both of us." With each massage, Lucy became steadily more confident.

From that time forward, Lucy massaged Zoe every day until she had to go back to work. Even then she or Michael, or sometimes both of them together, would massage Zoe in the evening when they got home from work.

Having massaged her baby every day, Lucy says that she can now tell when Zoe is relaxing to her touch and when she is tightening up. "I can read her body language much better and notice areas that seem more tight than other parts of the body," Lucy says.

Nicolas

From the time he was born, the parents of Nicolas, now thirteen months old, carried him in cloth slings. Nicolas' father, Jim, preferred to carry the baby on his back, while his mother, Marie, carried him in the front.

Like Zoe, the blond-haired, blue-eyed Nicolas was his parents' first child. He was born in a hospital with a rooming-in facility where he remained with his mother after her natural delivery and was nursed by her on demand. Marie continued to nurse Nicolas until he was about four months old, then easily weaned him to a bottle. His parents thought he was just about the brightest, most perfect baby ever born.

"Then when he was about eleven months old, bedtime bedlam began," Jim says. In spite of all their efforts, Nicolas seemed to get "higher" at night rather than more relaxed. He definitely did not want to go to bed, and once in bed, he would cry and demand attention repeatedly throughout the night.

For the first time, bedtime became one of the most unpleasant times for parents and baby alike. Gone were the relaxing "thank-goodness-the-baby-is-down" evenings. Jim despaired of ever again getting enough sleep and was tired and cranky at work. There were times when both parents wondered why they had once thought that having a baby was a good idea.

One Saturday while Jim was trying to tire out Nicolas in the heated swimming pool at the YMCA, a massage therapist told him about baby massage, and the desperate father decided he and Marie had nothing to lose by trying it. On the way to their Santa Monica home, Jim made a quick, impulsive detour and bought a book on baby massage and some massage oil at a local massage supply store.

Nicolas loved the massage from the very beginning.

"I think he thought it was another way to avoid going to bed," Marie says. It also gave Jim a quiet break in the evening, when he could begin to relax and even snooze a little, while Marie massaged Nicolas.

For Marie, massage provided a new bond to her baby. "Although our intention was simply to get Nicolas to go to sleep easier and stay asleep longer, the massages became almost like a meditation for me," she says. "I felt I was deeply connecting with his little body not just on the surface but beneath the skin, connecting with his whole being."

As time went on, the more Marie massaged Nicolas, the more she became attuned to and could feel differences in his body, areas that seemed tighter than others. Or areas that just seemed to need a little more touch.

"Some nights it seemed like his little legs were growing and lengthening beneath my fingers," she says. "It was an incredible experience, and after that first night I came to look forward to it. For me, it was another way of understanding him."

That first night Nicolas was drowsy and almost asleep by the time the massage was over. He went to bed easily and slept a little longer before awakening his parents during the night. Jim thought blessed relief was in sight, and he was right. One evening near the end of the first week of nightly massages, Nicolas toddled over to his mother with his blanket and the plastic bottle of massage oil.

> Hippocrates, the father of medicine, said that "the way to health is to have an aromatic bath and scented massage every day."

"I nearly cried, I was so thrilled," Marie said. "I knew it was a wonderful experience for me, but I didn't realize just how important it had become to Nicolas in one week." After that first week of massage, Nicolas began once again to sleep through the night.

"And we lived happily ever after," says Jim wryly.

Actually that isn't the end of the tale. When Jim, who is a devoted father, saw what an important experience massage was for Marie, he, too, decided that this might be a way to have a good, quiet time between father and son.

"We've had a lot of active time together, like when I take him swimming, or swing him in the air," Jim says, "but I didn't know too many good ways to have quiet time except when he was asleep and I was holding him. And Nicolas didn't know anything about that."

Although he still lets Marie do the evening massages, on weekends Jim likes to take over.

"Nicolas loves getting two massages a day on the weekend," Marie says. "He seems like he's a little more active during Jim's massage. He has a tiny fuzzy bear he likes to wave around, and he definitely does not want a nap." So Marie usually gives Nicolas his bath after Jim's massage, while Jim takes the nap.

"Nicolas does play more quietly after Jim's massage and his bath," Marie says. "I've heard some fathers say they didn't like their children until they got to be older, but I think massage is a great way for a father to start to connect with his child at an early age."

Jim concurs. "I believe that like Marie I know Nicolas better and in a different way now and that we have a special close time together. I don't know how long he will want to continue having me massage him as he grows older, but I hope he and I will always have something that is uniquely special between us, male-to-male, you know. I'd like to think our massages are laying the groundwork for some special, enduring connection," Jim says.

Andrew

Jill Vyse, president of the Canadian Chapter of the International Association of Infant Massage, and the director of a Canadian massage school, wrote us about her work with Andrew (not his real name), a three-year-old who had drowned and then was revived by rescue workers. The experience left him severely disabled physically and mentally.

Andrew protested loudly prior to, and cried during, each of his physiotherapy sessions. His mother and Jill began doing pediatric massage on his back and legs prior to the physiotherapy sessions in order to loosen muscle contractures and to ease the pain of the sessions.

"It became very clear that this little boy loved massage and was desperate to continue it, not to stop for physio," Jill writes. They began to use massage as a reward to follow the physiotherapy sessions, using the same blanket and the same lavender scented oil each time.

"There was a distinct decrease in crying, definite and measurable physical improvements, and very clear facial expressions—all of which were new for Andrew," Jill says.

Baby massage, for Andrew, has been therapeutic, pleasurable, and a highlight of his continuing efforts to recover.

Justin

Justin is the four-month-old son of Dave and Reina Johnson. Formerly a dentist in the Philippine Islands, Reina came to the United States in 1994, from her hometown of Pasig, near Manila.

After her arrival in the United States, she met Dave, a licensed psychiatric technician, and eventually they were married. Justin is their first child, and while she takes care of him, Reina studies for the dental board exams, which would allow her to practice dentistry in California.

Reina combines her knowledge of traditional Filipino methods of child care with books and magazines she read during her pregnancy. As a child, Reina herself was "exercised" and massaged by her mother much as she now does for Justin.

During her pregnancy, Reina massaged her belly and talked to her unborn baby. "Sometimes he would kick more when I was talking to him," she says.

In the Philippines, when a baby is about three weeks old, the mother begins to massage/exercise the baby. Reina demonstrated for us how while she is nursing Justin, she gently jiggles his legs and hands and rubs the top of his head.

"This helps him have a round head," she says, as she proudly displays Justin's beautifully rounded head.

Reina counts out loud in a delighted voice as she gently moves Justin's legs out straight and then back into his trunk, bending them up to his chest. She does the same as she moves his arms from his chest out straight, then back over his chest, and raises his arms up over his head and down again to his side. Justin smiles and coos, keeping his eyes on mother all the time.

"You're not pushing the baby," Reina stresses. "You're helping him get the idea of what to do with his legs and arms. You're moving them so he can feel the way he needs to move them."

Reina stresses that you must always be alert and sensitive to how your baby wants to move. As Justin's muscles developed, Reina moved to more advanced exercises. Now, almost as soon as she begins to pull him up by his arms, Justin straightens his back and stands upright.

"All of this also helps Justin exercise his energy because he doesn't yet know how to do it for himself," Reina says. "In the Philippines, when the baby can walk, women no longer continue the exercise/massage regime because now the child can work off his energy himself."

To bathe Justin, Reina does not put him in a tub filled with water. Rather she pours warm water over various parts of his body and as she does so, she rubs the water along that body part much as you would do if you were using oil.

> *Your participation as a parent is the key factor in your baby's emotional, spiritual, physical, and intellectual development.*

"All of this is play for the baby," she says, "but you, as the mother, have more in mind. You're helping this baby develop strong muscles and get ready to do his next movements."

Reina says that according to what she reads, Justin looks and acts like a six-month-old baby. She compares her baby to two others each born within a week of Justin, but whose mothers have not massaged/exercised their babies. She categorically affirms that they are not as well developed as Justin.

One of Justin's favorite games with daddy involves sitting in Dave's lap and, with Dave holding his arms, sliding backward down Dave's legs.

"There's always a way you can move and touch your baby," Reina says. "Here, Dave's knees massage Justin's back."

Sometimes Reina sings children's songs in Tagalog to Justin while she moves her hands down along his body, jiggling his sides or his back. Sometimes she uses her lips to jiggle his skin, getting sweet laughter from Justin.

"You can't touch new babies too much," Reina says.

We later learned from the proud parents that because he is so congenial and calm, and interacts so well with strangers, a talent agent has decided to represent Justin as one of his clients.

Penelope

Penelope, the daughter of parents we will call Irene and Michael, came to massage late in life. She was three-and-a-half when her new brother was born. While mother Irene was in the hospital, recovering from her delivery, a nurse showed her how to massage her newborn son.

"When I returned from the hospital," Irene says, "I had Penelope help me get the materials together to massage the baby and brought along some special new toys for Penelope."

Penelope stood near her mother, watching for a while before playing nearby, looking up frequently—ever vigilant as to what was happening. Once she looked up, frowning, and asked if the "wassage" would hurt the baby. Irene reassured her that it would not. Irene also recognized that Penelope's reversion to using "w's" instead of "m's" reflected some insecurity toward her place in the family.

As the nurse had instructed her, Irene talked to both the baby and Penelope while she was massaging the baby. She talked about how good the massage was feeling and how strong it was going to make the baby.

"This will make your legs grow strong and firm," she said as she massaged the baby's legs. Penelope wanted to massage the baby, and Irene helped her put oil on the newborn's feet and rub it around.

"You're making firm feet," her mother said, and Penelope laughed.

When she finished massaging the newborn, Irene asked Penelope if she would like a massage.

Penelope seemed pleased, but that first time she would only lie still long enough to have her legs and feet rubbed. Then she wanted to be up and about.

"She was so cute, prancing around, looking down at her legs every now and then," Irene says.

The next day when Irene got ready to massage the baby, Penelope wanted to be massaged first. Irene explained to her that she needed to massage the baby first, so he could go to sleep. Then she and Penelope could have their special massage together.

Irene got one of Penelope's dolls and suggested Penelope massage it while mother massaged her brother. That interested Penelope. Sitting beside her mother and watching her more alertly than the previous day, Penelope began to slather her doll with oil, explaining to it, "I wassaging my baby while mama's wassaging hers. Then mama will wassage me."

After both "babies" had been put down for their naps, Penelope allowed Irene to massage her entire body, except for her face.

As Penelope grew more used to the daily massage time, the two "mothers" fell into a routine. Penelope began helping Irene gather materials for the massage for both her brother and her doll. Sometimes she would massage the doll, sometimes she would just watch her mother. More and more, she just played quietly nearby. Also, like the baby, she was often so relaxed after her massage that she took her nap without protest, whereas when the baby first came home, Penelope was very demanding of her mother's time after the baby was asleep.

Irene believes that massage has benefitted both the new baby and Penelope, helping both be more relaxed and reassuring Penelope that there is still a special place for her in the family.

But baby massage isn't the only technique to help your baby become a brighter, happier, better adjusted child. In the chapters that follow we will look at other complementary techniques for giving your baby a good head start in life.

CHAPTER 5

The Mozart Effect
A Link to Baby Intelligence

We know that touch is extremely important to infants. But equally important are other types of stimulation you provide for your baby—practices that help babies maximize their intellectual potential. You, as the parent, play a key role in determining whether your baby's intellectual development will be simply average or above average. But what *type* of experiences should you be offering your baby? Several recent studies have proven an astonishing fact: *music* can enhance intelligence, and shape minds.

This phenomenon is called the "Mozart effect." Long suspected as being true, the beneficial effects of classical music were finally definitively proven by researchers at the University of California at Irvine in the mid-1990s. They found that undergraduates who listened to Mozart, specifically to Mozart's "Sonata for Two Pianos in D Major," scored better on a spatial IQ test. In another Irvine study preschool children were given piano keyboard training and after six months, they could play basic melodies by Mozart and Beethoven. They also exhibited dramatic improvement in such tests of spatial intelligence as solving puzzles and mazes, and drawing geometric figures, compared to children receiving computer lessons or other non-musical stimulation. The *kind* of music to

> Music can enhance intelligence and shape minds.

which students are exposed makes an enormous difference to the effect. Modern, minimalist scores or relaxing, easy listening music, or taped stories had far less dramatic impacts—indeed, in many cases, none—than did Mozart.

So what's so special about Mozart? Unlike other forms of music, Mozart has unique transforming properties. Its rhythm, its mathematical elegance which combines complexity and clarity, stimulates the body's autonomic nervous system and rewires brain cell connections. Mozart's music provides feelings of well-being, develops brain connections needed for higher-order thinking, and even has healing properties. Dr. Gordon Shaw, one of the researchers, suggests that Mozart's music may "warm up" the brain through symmetries and patterns that enhance thinking and reasoning. He likens the Mozart effect to an "internal language of higher brain function" and believes we are all born with the ability to process music in a fairly sophisticated manner.

Actor Gerard Depardieu can personally testify to the beneficial effects of Mozart. Before Depardieu enjoyed success in the art of oratory he suffered from a severe stuttering problem. He sought help from the Tomatis Center in Paris, an ear, nose, and throat clinic where he was given Mozart to listen to for two hours a day. After only a few days he experienced noticeable improvements in his speech and overall health, and after a few months was able to speak clearly.

A study at Cornell University reinforces the importance of the Mozart effect for babies. Four-month-old babies were played segments of pieces by Mozart. The pieces were then broadcast in a jumbled format. The babies became irritable during the jumbled music, but were calm and happy with Mozart in the original.

Listening to classical music, in general, acts as a sort of "exercise" for improving concentration and enhancing thinking abilities. Dr. Gordon Shaw believes that music taps into the inherent structure of the brain, and early music training could exercise the brain's inherent ability to form patterns and enhance spatial reasoning, useful for higher mathematics and reasoning in science.

Providing this "exercise" for your baby will help shape the neurological connections in your baby's brain and directly improve your baby's intellec-

THE MOZART EFFECT

tual growth, especially in music and mathematics.

Having your baby *listen* to classical music is extremely beneficial, but early exposure to music lessons may be *even better* for your child's intellectual growth. Researchers at the University of Konstanz in Germany examined the brains of nine string musicians using MRI technology. They found that in all the musicians the section of the brain used for fingering the stringed instruments was much larger compared to that of nonmusicians. They found the difference in brain matter was due to the *age* when the musicians started playing their instruments, not the number of hours spent playing them. So early music exposure can change the capacity of the brain in favor of musical ability. The other interesting factor here is the apparent connection between exposure to classical music and improved mathematical ability—and that exposure can begin even before your child is born.

Recent research and medical discoveries have made it clear that babies are born with predispositions to learn and understand certain information. Some of these predispositions are genetic, others might actually be learned *in utero*. There is some evidence that babies exposed to Mozart by their mothers during pregnancy might be predisposed to have greater musical or mathematical potential. Studies reveal that when the brain receives outside stimulation, its physical structure changes. Research also indicates

Savvy Statesmen

The link between music and enhanced brain development in infants has not only been discovered by researchers and new mothers, it was recognized by former Georgia governor Zell Miller. Every mother in Georgia now leaves the hospital with a classical music tape or CD. Miller told parents, "Einstein knew it. So did Galileo. They knew that there was a direct relationship between music and math." He suggested parents should give their children a "smart start," especially in "the spatial, temporal reasoning that underlies math and engineering," by playing classical music for them early and often, affirming that research "shows a link between classical music and the enhanced brain development of infants" and "links the study of music to better school performance and higher scores on college entrance exams." The Georgia tape has selections from Beethoven, Mozart, Handel, Schubert, Vivaldi, and Bach. Similarly the Florida legislature passed a "Beethoven Babies" amendment requiring state child-care facilities to play classical music every day.

that the experiences we provide our babies, in the womb and out, through nutrition and physical and mental exercises—listening to Mozart in particular—will affect how well they understand, reason, and remember. The emerging stark fact is shocking: the type of experience you provide for your baby *in utero* and in her early years is more important for your child's intellectual potential than what she might do in junior high school or later.

Prenatal Mozart

Don Campbell, author of *The Mozart Effect*, describes how prenatal exposure to Mozart can have lifelong beneficial effects on health and behavior, can improve thinking, strengthen creativity, and relieve stress. Even in the womb, babies develop a taste for certain sounds, melodies, and tempos. They seem to respond to the pacing and complexity of Mozart—and it may even sharpen their memory.

In the 1950s and 1960s, Alfred Tomatis, a French physician and ear specialist, studied the effects of music on babies in the womb and describes in his book, *The Conscious Ear*, how the unborn baby is capable of hearing a fairly broad range, and after birth can retain memory of the sounds. He called Mozart's music "liberating, curative, and healing."

Gregorian Chant or Rock and Roll?

One of Dr. Alfred Tomatis's most interesting discoveries was when he was invited to a monastery in the South of France. He was asked to investigate and cure a mysterious malady—a sort of monk's version of yuppie flu—that had overcome a group of Benedictine monks. Dr. Tomatis could find nothing physically wrong with the monks, and nothing wrong with their diet or environment. What he did find is that the monks had—as a result of Vatican II reforms—cut back on their daily chanting.

When the monks resumed their old schedule of chanting—under doctor's orders—they found their health restored. Some have called this variation of the Mozart effect "sonic healing." However it works, the physical power of music has been recognized by every culture in the world—from the Zulus of South Africa whose most important ceremonies are full of drumming and singing, to contemporary Japan where one can buy classical music CDs that claim to cure specific ailments (for headaches, Mendelssohn's "Spring Song," Dvorak's "Humoresque," and George Gershwin's "American in Paris" are recommended), to the ancient Greek philosopher Plato who thought music was the most important and—because of its power for good or ill—the most dangerous of the arts. Plato's observation has been confirmed in our own time by cities—such as the city of Edmonton in Alberta, Canada—that have piped classical music into public parks and noticed a resulting dramatic fall in reported crimes, including drug-dealing, and in lowered aggression among pedestrians.

So choosing the right music for your baby—classical music or spiritually uplifting music like Gregorian chant—is crucial. Aside from the highly negative cultural influences to be found in much popular music, the repetitive throbbing of rock unlike the complexity of classical music—might actually wire the brain in ways that are harmful to future learning, the very reverse of the complexity that links classical music to mathematics.

We know, in fact, that in plant studies, classical music improves plant growth and flowering, while rock stunts it; and that babies in the womb show a strong preference for classical music (and can remember it, and respond to familiar pieces after they are born) than to rock, which causes fetal irritability.

Some doctors even assert that Americans now live in a "toxic" culture: too noisy and full of stress; over-mechanized, thereby discouraging physical exercise; full of unhealthy, processed foods; and bombarded by a media driven by its audience's insatiable appetite for lust and violence.

So the next time you turn on the radio, watch television, or play a CD, think about what your baby will be absorbing—and how your baby might be influenced positively or negatively. It might be time to put away the Stones's *Voodoo Lounge* and play Mozart's *Eine Kleine Nachtmusik*. The change might be soothing, healing, and strengthening for both you and your baby.

Parents who have used the Mozart effect for their unborn babies can testify to its effectiveness. Beth and Paul of Tampa, Florida, played Mozart for their three-month-old daughter. During the late stages of pregnancy, Beth played Mozart for her daughter by pressing small speakers attached to an audio belt—the sort of thing you might wear if you were to use a Walkman while jogging—against her stomach. "I really sense she recognizes the Mozart. She'll stop and listen... her eyes widen."

Some Chicago hospitals have been using the Mozart effect in their neonatal units, not only for its intelligence-enhancing elements but also for its healing properties, with positive results. One baby girl was born prematurely with a life-threatening condition. Doctors put her on life support with little hope of survival. The only positive stimulation she received was from constant infusions of Mozart that nurses piped into the neonatal unit at the request of the little girl's mother. Until the age of three the girl's motor skills were very poor, but she tested far ahead of her years in abstract reasoning. One evening, her parents took her to a chamber music concert. For days afterward, she pretended to play the violin using an empty paper towel tube and a chopstick. When her mother enrolled her in violin lessons, she proved to be an incredible child prodigy. She not only produced recognizable musical sounds from the violin immediately, but the sounds corresponded to classical pieces she played from memory.

> Mozart's music provides feelings of well-being, develops brain connections needed for higher-order thinking, and even has healing properties.

The easiest way to play music for your unborn baby is by using headphones. Place the headphones on your stomach for your baby to listen. Adjust the volume to your preference, but it does not have to be—indeed, should not be—too loud. If you don't have headphones you can listen to music through your home or car speakers. It is more difficult for your baby to hear but the music can still provide stimulation. Play music for your baby whenever it is convenient for both of you. Continue playing music for your baby after she is born. Remember, the stimulative experiences you provide for your baby during her first months will determine how competent, capable, and creative your child will become.

Comparing Composers for Your Child

In deciding which classical music to play, here are some ready guidelines.

First, any selections from Mozart are indisputably the best. The evidence supporting the Mozart Effect is the best-documented and most wide-ranging. Some of the odder evidence includes a monastery in Brittany that found that cows exposed to Mozart produce more milk.

In Japan, the Ohara Brewery has discovered that playing Mozart in its yeast rooms increases yeast-density by a factor of ten, making for better sake. Perhaps more relevant to your baby is that Washington State has discovered that playing Mozart for Asian immigrants in English-as-a-Second-Language courses speeds up the immigrants' ability to learn English.

So the bottom line is, play Mozart for your child.

But for the sake of diversity, you might want some other composers to choose from. Here's a helpful list of good alternatives.

- The three B's—Bach, Beethoven, and Brahms
- Tchaikovsky (young children might particularly enjoy "The 1812 Overture")
- Vivaldi
- Handel
- Haydn
- Rachmaninoff
- Schubert
- Chopin (especially for young babies)
- Sibelius ("Finlandia" is good for boys who love it when you read them adventures stories—it *sounds* like adventure)
- Aaron Copland (especially "Rodeo," which young children like to dance to, and "Appalachian Spring")
- The Strauss Waltzes (once your child can walk, she can waltz—the precise steps teach coordination, discipline, and are good way for parent and child to bond)

And don't neglect the traditional children's classics:

- Benjamin Britten's "The Young Person's Guide to the Orchestra"
- Rimsky-Korsakov's "The Flight of the Bumblebee"
- Prokofiev's "Peter and the Wolf" and "The Love of Three Oranges"
- "The Light Cavalry Overture," by Franz von Suppe
- "The William Tell Overture" and "The Barber of Seville," by Rossini
- "A Night on Bald Mountain" and "The Great Gate of Kiev," by Modest Mussorgsky
- The marches of Edward Elgar and John Philip Sousa
- "The Planets," the "Suite Number One in E-Flat" and "Suite Number Two in F," by Gustav Holst
- "The Folk Song Suite," by Vaughn Williams

An Operatic Beginning for Baby

Don't forget that Mozart wrote operas as well, and that opera is a great way not only to expose your child to wonderful music, but to foreign languages—including French, German, and Italian—a Mozart Effect "twofer." Young children might particularly enjoy Mozart's "Magic Flute." Many young children respond better to singing—they like the sound of the human voice—than they do to music alone.

The great thing about opera, if you're expecting, is to remember this: *your baby has the potential to learn any language, and the best time to start may be before she's born.* Sound surprising? It is but less so as we learn more and more about how quickly unborn babies develop and how sensitive they are to stimulation, especially to sound.

Just as an unborn baby can hear her mother's voice, or benefit from the Mozart Effect, so too can she be exposed to foreign languages, especially as "sweetened" with music, as in opera, with this immediate benefit: the sounds and word patterns will not seem foreign to your baby.

Babies very quickly begin associating certain sounds as definable speech and language. They also *reject* sounds that do not fit a linguistic grid that is established very early in life.

The best time to begin language training for your child is before she's six months of age, and you can begin while your baby is still in the womb.

You will notice, as your baby develops, that she quickly learns to *discriminate* between sounds made by the people around her—she may look confused at a stranger's voice or someone with a low, booming voice, while showing immediate recognition and happiness at the sound of her mother's soft, lilting voice. Some of this recognition—for parents's voices, for music, for what language is "foreign" and what language is not—is begun *in utero*. So put on your CD of "Madame Butterfly" and start your child on the road to learning good music *and* a foreign language.

Mommy as Diva

Don't neglect singing to your baby—when she's in the womb and after she's born.

If you're self-conscious about your singing, do what nonsinging actors do when they're signed up for a musical performance—talk your way through. Talk to your baby every chance you get. Remember: Your baby loves interacting with you. She thrives on it.

Talk to your baby as if she understands every word you are saying. Just think out loud. If you take your baby on a walk describe everything around to your baby; as you perform tasks around the house tell your baby about what you are doing—or sing about it.

At massage time or bath time (a perfect venue for singing) continue your "one-sided" conversation. Obviously your baby won't be able to understand every word, but by speaking to her you are providing her with the sounds, rhythm, and patterns of language.

The more your baby absorbs your speech sounds, the more her sounds will start replicating real language. As your baby becomes accustomed to a particular language with its rhythm of sounds, she will go on to use that language. During this early "language forming" stage, before she is six months old, is the best time to start introducing a foreign language.

It is best if you speak the foreign language yourself or, through simple memorization, can sing an aria in Italian.

Second best is to play tapes, preferably opera tapes (much more interesting for little ears than adult "learning language" tapes). But another alternative is foreign language tapes designed for children, especially tapes that go along with picture books. After age three your child's ability to learn a second language declines as she becomes "deaf" to sounds other than her native tongue.

New discoveries in the language abilities of preborns and newborns are causing school administrators to rethink the conventional method of waiting until junior high or high school to introduce a second language. But as the schools move slowly, you could give your baby a real head start.

Your baby's brain is like a sponge taking in everything around her, so be mindful of what she is absorbing. Your baby will not only pick up on your speech, but also your tone and temperament when speaking, which is why song can be so helpful, because it generally ensures that you will be animated and happy.

Mothers seem to have a natural instinct to sing and talk to their babies. Follow that instinct. You should read books aloud, pray aloud, and sing to your baby—starting while you're pregnant. Fathers, brothers, sisters, and other family members should also talk or sing to your baby. All of this will stimulate her brain to work, react, and grow.

Remember, every baby is different and some develop language abilities sooner than others. But keep singing and talking to your baby. It is a baby's natural inclination to talk, and if you keep at it, clearly and consistently, your baby *will* develop superb language abilities.

CHAPTER 6

Brain Development in the Womb and Out

From the moment of conception your child has been given all the genetic material she needs to develop as a unique individual. But that does not mean that your unborn baby doesn't need all the help you can provide *before* she is born.

Your baby is dependent on you for proper nutrition. But she is also dependent on you for her prenatal experiences that might help shape her potential once she is born.

We have already examined how the Mozart Effect can help babies while they are still in the womb. But there are additional forms of prenatal stimulation that seem to have a favorable effect on infant intelligence, and help babies and mothers bond.

The most effective way to stimulate your baby and enhance her brain development while still in the womb is through sound, and not just through music, but through your own voice.

All of your baby's senses have been formed and are active by the fifth month of pregnancy. Hearing starts a bit earlier. The internal parts of the ear are formed in the first eight weeks, and two weeks later, the outer ear will have formed. At approximately sixteen weeks your baby can hear your voice while she is still in the womb. The verbal bond between mother and baby can be, generally is, and should be, formed now, *in utero*.

Just as the heart beats in your unborn baby's body—and can sometimes be heard as early as twelve weeks after conception—the brain is functional as well. At two months after conception your baby's brain is already receiving stimulation and even providing its own by the physical control it exerts over swallowing, changing position, sucking, kicking, or touching (your baby's sense of touch begins developing now). By the fourth month, the tangible effect of baby's touch and activity is mutual. This is when many mothers start feeling their baby move.

Many couples find, at this stage, that very gentle stroking of a mother's abdomen is relaxing for them, and a good start to the bonding process that allows a father's involvement. Put on some relaxing classical music—remember that your baby can be disturbed by loud or discordant noises—and enjoy a light, stroking massage. Talk softly to your baby about all your hopes and dreams for her. Even make it a romantic and nutritious night-time activity, with a bowl of strawberries or other fruit (which is good for you and your baby), and a bowl of honey to dip them in nearby. As your pregnancy develops, you might want your husband to expand the massage to cover your tired back, swollen ankles, or other problem areas. Whatever you do, never forget to gently stroke your abdomen, and speak or sing to the baby inside.

> The most effective way to stimulate your baby and enhance her brain development while still in the womb is through sound.

Your participation as a parent is the key factor in your baby's emotional, spiritual, physical, and intellectual development. And constant communication with your child, starting prenatally, is vitally important. Your baby craves stimulation. Even when she is still in the womb she is affected by what goes on outside. Stimulation of your unborn baby's senses, through proper nutrition, through loving speech to your unborn child, through stroking your abdomen, or through the Mozart Effect, can shape the development of a child's growing brain.

Think of your baby's brain as a smooth surface that becomes grooved with ridges as the baby absorbs information. Beneath that smooth surface lies your baby's invaluable genetic inheritance. That is a given. But the potential use your baby makes of that inheritance can be shaped. You can provide her with valuable experiences contributing to the development of intelligence and creativity.

It was once thought that a child's memory begins at age three. The evidence for this was anecdotal. That was as far back as most adults could remember. But new studies in early child development have found that babies learn and remember from the time their senses are formed in the womb. In other words, even though many adults cannot *remember* experiences unless they happened after age three, our brains are absorbing most of their information and stimuli *before* age three. Babies obviously have keen memories, for this is how they learn, and never is learning more important than in the early months and years of a child's life when the mental blueprint is engraved for that child's potential.

At five months *in utero* your baby's brain will have developed all the brain cells it ever will. Your child's brain will almost cease to grow after three years of age, so stimulating your baby during this "brain molding" window-of-opportunity is an important step to ensuring your baby's optimal intellectual growth.

Babies' Brain Development Chart

10-18 weeks in utero	Total number of brain cells formed
32 weeks in utero	Brain doubles in weight
Birth	Brain reaches 25% of its adult weight
2 months	Motor-control areas of the brain develop (baby can reach and grab objects)
4 months	Depth perception and binocular vision refined
6 months	Brain reaches 50% of its adult weight
1 year	Brain reaches 70% of its adult weight. Speech areas of brain develop (baby says first words)
20 weeks in utero to 2 years	Brain's learning phase. Brain cells increase in size
3 years	Brain reaches more than 90 percent of maximum size

Your Baby's Brain Development

Even though your baby at five months *in utero* has all the brain cells she will ever have, most of the brain cells are not yet "wired" or organized to perform many of what could be your child's intellectual talents. It is through the stimulative experiences she encounters from five months *in utero* to age two that will put the brain cells "in order." This learning phase is your "window" to make a difference in your baby's intelligence. During this phase, your baby's brain becomes "electrified" with energy as it is bombarded with new stimuli. In fact, by age two, your baby's brain has twice as many synapses and uses up twice as much energy as yours! Every time your baby hears classical music, reaches for a soft teddy bear, or watches a colorful jack-in-the-box, circuits of "electricity" fire through the brain, organizing brain cells and wiring them for different functions. You will witness the exciting results of this brain activity as your baby smiles at you for the first time, utters her first word, or takes her first step.

What wires your baby's brain is the experiences you give her. The more synapses or brain messages that occur in your baby's brain, the brighter your baby will be. Your baby's early experiences determine which brain cells are used, how the circuits of the brain will be wired, and, perhaps, the ultimate intellectual potential of your baby.

Your baby's IQ comes down to *you*. You as the parent are your baby's most important teacher. The key to having a brighter baby is being attentive to your baby's needs. Educating your baby does not require elaborate technology, just attention—playing games, talking to her, baby massage, playing classical music, spending time with your baby. The key is hands-on parenting—finding time to provide stimulating experiences for your baby, which can be as simple as inviting her to touch a furry kitten or smell an apple pie baking in the oven.

And speaking of apple pie, let's look at how you can actually *feed* your baby's developing brain, starting while she's in the womb.

CHAPTER 7

Baby Intelligence and Mother's Diet

Touch, massage, and music for a brighter baby all have a common denominator: stimulation. The close bond you create with your baby and your attentiveness to her needs, especially during her first few years, dictates the intellectual growth your baby will have. Nutrition is yet another area in which you can provide the right kind of intellectual environment for your baby.

Pregnancy is the most unique and special time in a woman's life. There is no closer relationship between two people than between a mother and her unborn child. Even though the tiny human being is growing and developing into an individual, she still shares, among other things, the mother's nutrients and depends on her for sustenance. Surprisingly, a baby's learning and memory begin at this time.

As your baby breathes and swallows amniotic fluid while in the womb she becomes familiar with your diet. Foods that you eat break down and pass through the placenta to your baby. The chemical compounds unique to your body are also present in breastmilk. Studies have shown that babies already know and prefer their own mother's milk through exposure to the mother's chemical compounds while in the womb. If you abruptly change your diet while pregnant, your baby will notice! She may become confused by the change and may not be able to recognize your breastmilk after birth.

Breastmilk and IQ

Several new studies suggest that there is a link between breast-feeding babies and children with higher IQ. One 1998 study that appeared in the *Journal of Pediatrics* tracked more than 1,000 children in New Zealand through the age of 18. The study showed that those children who were breast-fed as babies did better in school and scored higher on standardized tests in mathematics and reading. The conclusion? Fatty acids that are present in breast milk but not in formula promote lasting brain development.

> The best way to acquire optimum brain function for you and your baby is to have a balanced, healthy diet and lifestyle.

Fatty acids are essential to building brain cells and are also present in fish—(replete with omega-3 fatty acids)—which is why fish is popularly called "brain food." Don't be concerned about the word "fat." We are talking about "good fat" as opposed to "bad fat." "Good fat," from such foods as olive oil, nuts, and fish (the best are salmon and tuna) is actually necessary for a balanced, healthy diet, and will promote better breastmilk for your baby—and better intelligence. Some other intelligence-enhancing elements in breastmilk are lactose, or milk sugar, which is directly related to brain growth; lecithin, which assists in the formation of brain tissue; and taurine, an amino acid. Preemies who were fed formulas without this important element, taurine, experienced learning difficulties.

So respond to your baby's needs. Nature has designed your milk especially for your baby—it has all the essential food elements your baby needs for optimum brain growth and IQ.

Increase the Zinc, Folic Acid, and Iron

We have long known the benefits for pregnant mothers of taking extra vitamins and minerals—prenatal vitamins are now routinely prescribed by doctors. But recently doctors have been recommending extra zinc and especially folic acid in a mother's diet. A recent study from the University of Alabama-Birmingham shows that babies whose mothers took zinc while pregnant were bigger, were born later (that is, more fully developed and mature), had a lower risk of infection, and had bigger head sizes. After your baby is born, she will absorb zinc from breastmilk better than from cow's milk or formula, and zinc is important for proper growth.

But how does this relate to intelligence? Recent studies have shown that babies who are very underweight and fail to grow properly can also suffer impaired intelligence. Studies have linked babies with larger head sizes to increased intelligence.

How much zinc should you take when pregnant? The University of Alabama-Birmingham study showed beneficial results when pregnant women were getting up to 38 milligrams of zinc in their diet—higher than the government's recommended 15 milligrams per day. However, most doctors agree that 19 milligrams for lactating mothers during the first six months, and 16 milligrams during the second six months are sufficient amounts. Of course, you should eat a balanced diet while pregnant, but, with your doctor's consent, it is perfectly safe to take a zinc supplement throughout your pregnancy. Try getting zinc into your daily diet from some natural sources such as seafood (especially oysters), lean meat, poultry, eggs, legumes, and whole-grain foods.

Recent studies have also found that babies whose mothers got enough folic acid during the early weeks of pregnancy reduced the risk of brain and spinal cord defects by half. Few, if any, supplements offer more dramatic benefits than that. But the good news is that you can get most or all of your folic acid requirement naturally. If you eat a well-balanced diet of three to five daily servings of vegetables (especially green leafy ones like spinach) and two to four daily servings of fruit (oranges, strawberries, and bananas are good sources), you should meet your optimum folic acid intake. All prenatal vitamins contain folic acid, as do legumes and most cereals. See your doctor about the right level for you, but 1,000 micrograms a day is generally regarded as the maximum safe dose.

Iron is another essential mineral for mother and baby, and most pregnant women need a supplement to get as much as they need. Especially in the last trimester, your baby will be storing iron from your iron supply. So be sure to include iron rich foods—like prunes and prune juice, apricots, whole grains, and lean beef—in your diet and be sure your prenatal vitamin includes iron, as well as zinc and folic acid.

Vitamin B-12

Getting enough of vitamin B-12 when you are breastfeeding is important for your baby's brain and spinal cord development. A deficiency of B-12 in breastmilk can lead to brain and spinal cord damage in a growing baby. Vitamin B-12 acts with folic acid to form and strengthen cells, promote growth and development, protect nerve endings, and prevent nerve damage. Vitamin B-12 also produces acetylcholine, a neurotransmitter that enhances brain function, especially memory and learning. Even though your body can store B-12 for a long period of time, it is important for you, if you are breastfeeding, to consume it during your nursing months in order for the vitamin to be present in your breastmilk. If your diet includes milk and dairy products, an abundant source of B-12, you probably don't have to worry about having a deficiency. Other sources for B-12 are eggs, yeast, and seafood. If you are a strict vegetarian you will have a harder time getting B-12 into your diet because it is not found in most fruits or vegetables. But soybeans and soybean products, sea vegetables, alfalfa, and hops have trace amounts. Check with your doctor to be sure you are getting enough B-12 in your diet.

"Smart" Herbs

Sometimes the old ways are best. That sounds like something your mother or grandmother would say, but it is good advice, because when it comes to promoting optimum health and healing *sometimes* the old ways, the *natural* ways, are best. Throughout many cultures, including early American culture, herbs were prescribed not only as remedies for various illnesses and ailments, but as a part of general good health and nutrition. Today, many alternative nutritionists prescribe echinacea for colds or ear aches; garlic supplements as a general antibiotic; chamomile to fight pain or, along with mint, to settle an upset stomach; or calendula as a salve for skin irritations. There might even be herbs that can help the brain.

The best way to acquire optimum brain function for you and your baby is to have a balanced, healthy diet and lifestyle. Overall, a healthy mother means a healthy baby. There are some nutritional supplements that have a long history of use as brain nutrients. But some herbal remedies can be dangerous or even life-threatening so always consult your doctor before introducing anything "new" to your body and your baby's body.

A Sweetener to Avoid

The jury is still out on the definite side effects of aspartame sweetener, better known as Nutrasweet, approved by the FDA for wide use in 1981. But a study done at the Children's Hospital in Boston found that mothers who ingest aspartame while pregnant may be putting their unborn babies at risk for decreased mental capacity and intelligence. Some infants (possibly one in ten) lack an enzyme that breaks down an amino acid called phenylalanine, an ingredient in aspartame. Phenylalanine is passed through the mother's placenta to her baby whenever she eats or drinks something with aspartame. Aspartame is now found in a multitude of sugar-free, low-fat foods including carbonated and uncarbonated beverages, cereals, desserts, and chewing gum. So if you have to drink that soda, better check the label first for aspartame.

Alcohol, Cigarettes, Caffeine, and Drugs

Some other things to avoid while you are pregnant are alcohol, cigarettes, caffeine, and drugs. Remember, anything you take into your body is passed on to your baby via the placenta. The chemicals in alcohol and cigarettes, for example, may be only slightly damaging to you but toxic to your baby. Consuming these substances while pregnant could alter your baby's developing brain function, stunting your baby's IQ. It is better to think *naturally* when it comes to your diet and your baby.

But remember that if herbs can cure like drugs do, they should be treated with the same caution. For this reason, it's best to avoid apparently anodyne things like herbal tea unless you have your doctor's consent—and even then, be sure not to overdo. Some herbal teas are perfectly safe, but it depends on the totality of their ingredients. When in doubt, skip it.

It's also best to skip caffeine. If you have "morning sickness" you will probably want to skip morning coffee anyway—the very smell of it might make you feel nauseated.

While caffeine can be bad for your baby—think of how easily you get "overcaffeinated," and then think of what the effects might be on your child—recent studies have shown that a moderate caffeine intake of no more than two cups of tea, coffee, or soda is probably okay.

If you do choose to drink coffee, tea, or soda, the best bet is tea. Sodas can contain potentially dangerous sweeteners or can be full of wasteful calories from sugar. Coffee can pack too much of a caffeine punch for many pregnant mothers, raising your blood pressure (and your baby's) and increasing your stress level. But recent studies have shown that tea—both green tea and black tea—might actually promote good health. A cup of tea that's drunk within an hour of its steeping is full of health-promoting antioxidants that protect the body from "free radicals"—unstable molecules that destroy healthy tissues. The even better news about tea is that the antioxidants are present in both caffeinated and *decaffeinated* tea. So try decaffeinated first and see if the flavor is enough. If you still need a caffeine boost, think of turning your soda fix or coffee habit into tea time—and make it a special and relaxing time.

Alcohol is another forbidden drink, though some doctors are prepared to wink at an occasional *single* glass of wine or beer. In England, nursing mothers in hospitals are even allowed the dark, rich beer, Guinness Stout, which is thought to have useful nutrients and help relax a nursing mother, easing her milk flow.

But *all* alcohol consumption carries risks, the most common for your baby being lower birth weight. Some of the risks—as seen in "Fetal Alcohol Syndrome"—can be severe. It is safest not to drink at all while you're pregnant. But whatever your choice, don't do it in ignorance. Consult your doctor first, and abide by his advice.

Smoking is perhaps the most widely discouraged legal drug of all. Smoking while pregnant is like standing behind an idling car and breathing in the fumes—it's bad for you and bad for your baby, raising the risks of miscarriage or premature birth. Smoking can also complicate the reactions of the unborn baby to caffeine or alcohol exposure. If you've ever needed one last reason to give up smoking, your baby should be it.

As for drugs, even prescription drugs or over-the-counter drugs need to be approved by your doctor. Common medicines—like aspirin—can complicate a pregnancy. So ask your doctor before you take any drug.

As for other, illicit drugs, the answer is to give them up now—if not for your own well-being, than for your child's. There is direct evidence that mothers who ingest cocaine and other illicit drugs during pregnancy put their children at risk: they can even be born addicted to drugs, their health is more fragile, they are more likely to score poorly on intelligence tests, and the mothers are, obviously, less well able to take care of their young. Pregnant women who take illegal drugs are committing child abuse through the umbilical cord. Don't do it. If you need help to kick an illegal drug habit—get it. Now.

> A healthy mother means a healthy baby.

The Basics of Good Nutrition for a Smart Child, a Strong Child

The nutritional key to building your baby's brain *in utero* is to eat "smart," and that means adopting a lifestyle that incorporates good nutrition and moderate exercise.

A good diet for a pregnant or lactating mother would include 2300 calories with most of those—six to eleven servings a day—coming from carbohydrates: breads, cereals, rice, and pastas. Your next largest source of calories should come from fruits (especially vitamin-packed oranges and strawberries) and vegetables (broccoli, tomatoes, and spinach are the best, though some mothers find tomatoes too acidic for queasy stomachs, or that broccoli causes gas), about three to five servings of each. Two to three servings of dairy products will ensure you have the calcium you need for you and your baby (try always to have a glass or two of skim milk every day), and another two to three servings of lean meat, dried beans, lean poultry, fish, or nuts, will ensure your protein supply (you'll need about seventy-five to one hundred grams of protein).

Avoid desserts, pastries, and saturated fats. If you simply have to indulge, spring for a dessert that includes other nutrients you need—have a strawberry shortcake or make a sweet potato pie (sweet potatoes are a good source of vitamin A).

Don't worry about gaining weight during pregnancy. As long as you live according to your doctor's guidelines, get the exercise you need, and eat healthfully, you should be fine. Most mothers should gain about thirty pounds when they're pregnant with a single baby. So eat "smart," but do eat. Now is not the time to diet. And if you eat the right foods, and lead a healthy lifestyle, the good news is—you probably won't have to.

CHAPTER 8

Brain Exercises for Your Baby

For the first month, your baby will receive stimulation enough just by being with you and getting used to life outside the womb. This is a period to simply enjoy your baby, to share with your spouse all the joys of parenting, to trust your instincts and merely love your new bundle of joy.

It's best not to do too much this early on. For one thing, you will be recuperating from having given birth. For another, your child needs time to adapt to her new world, her eyes are not yet fully developed, and certain capacities, like speech, are difficult to rush, though you can set a tremendous foundation for growth.

You can help your baby feel at home by establishing a comforting routine. Spend plenty of time touching, cuddling, and massaging your child. This will help with bonding and with your child's sense of comfort, putting her at ease. Also, the Mozart Effect can be introduced immediately, but be sure to play the music softly. Too much stimulation, and too many loud noises, can disturb the baby or frighten her and do more harm than good.

You can also introduce toys, especially soft, cuddly ones that help stimulate a child's sense of touch, that are safe, that are not threatening, and that, again, can provide comfort, especially at nap times when your baby might want to hold on to something—but you might not want it to be you.

It's also a good time to talk to your child. Don't expect your child to be building her vocabulary, but she will be learning the basis of language, how sound becomes speech, and will be as responsive to your voice as she is to your touch.

It's important to remember, too, that all babies are different—that each is born an individual with her own predispositions, her own internal learning clock. Not all babies learn every skill at the same rate, and whether they start quickly or slowly is not necessarily any indication of future ability.

Much learning is, of course, done beneath the surface. The quiet watchful baby can be learning just as much as the active, talkative baby.

> Stereos equipped with display units—with lights that rise and fall with the pulse of the music—can provide useful visual stimulation to go with the aural stimulation. Try this once your baby is about three months old, when her range of sight extends to more than ten feet away.

So remember that some of the most important rules of parenting are: be calm, be patient, and be prepared to cope happily with every new challenge (from soiled diapers, to spilled food, to sleepless nights, to the extra time it takes to go anywhere when you need to pack your baby bag) that a new child brings.

Every parent in history—and there have been quite a lot of us—has been through this, and every child is naturally programmed in the womb to come into this world ready to explore, learn, and love. As a responsible parent, your role is to encourage your child, and provide the support and nurturing she needs to get a head start in life. And of course, if you ever have any questions, always consult your pediatrician.

The First Month

One of the first stimulators you can acquire for your child is a mobile that she can bat from her crib. She will benefit from examining the shapes, following their movement, examining their designs (and eventually colors), exercising her hand-eye (and hand-leg) coordination, and enjoying the music (if your mobile is so equipped).

Because young babies are themselves pretty much *immobile*, take advantage of having a captive audience and give your baby a play rug that is colorful, with geometric designs, and perhaps with toys attached that she can manipulate with her still developing fingers and grasping reflex.

You can also gently rock her in a baby rocker (or baby seat) while playing some soothing classical music.

The one crucial thing now, and later in your baby's life, is to interact with your child. Basic interactive games between parent and baby—like "peek-a-boo" or "this little piggy went to market" or having your baby track a finger that becomes a tickling "bee" or even shaking a rattle that you then give to your baby to shake—are the building blocks of a newborn's learning. Don't neglect them. Most important, don't miss the fun of these early weeks of your baby's life.

Babies, from their time in the womb, are continually absorbing or reacting to stimuli but can only express themselves, after they're born, through chortling baby noises until they're about one-and-a-half years old, when verbal language actually starts to develop. But just as babies can pick up the foundations of verbal languages quickly, so too will they learn your mannerisms and begin adopting your unconscious sign language. Your gestures can even help your child master the learning of speech and words.

Psychologists at the University of California and California State University have found that babies are able to learn gestures that, if reinforced by parents, will speed up a baby's ability to talk and stimulate intellectual development. The gestures do not have to be *formal* sign language. They can include waving, clapping, or any gesture that corresponds to a word. Try singing a song to your baby using gestures (for example "I'm a little teapot short and stout..."). By linking gestures and sounds during a baby's "pre-speech" phase, your baby will become excited about learning new gestures and, eventually, language.

Two Months

By about six weeks you'll get one of the biggest rewards a parent is given—your baby will smile at you. The interaction you've begun with your child from birth will now pay huge dividends as you and your baby make faces at each other and your baby learns to show emotions. Your baby is starting to become *social* and is learning to gain control of her body, especially her hands. She can even begin a modest exercise program to build her muscle tone and learn more about how to use her body.

Be sure to give your baby soft toys that have large geometrical designs—including spots, lines, or happy faces—that will stimulate both her tactile and visual senses.

Take advantage of her new sociability to increase your "quality time" with her, talking, singing, and playing simple games. Your baby will now start to "talk" back to you.

Three Months

Now your baby will turn active, and more vigorous exercises can begin to improve your baby's hand-eye coordination—for example, place a loose fitting cap on her head and have her take it off and wave it, or teach her to remove her socks.

Be sure to respond to every baby sound your baby makes. Talk to her as though the sounds are a legitimate conversation. By encouraging her, you will help make it happen.

Your baby will also be getting her first stirrings of independence. Give the baby some time to play and explore on her own. Let her experiment with early, attempted crawling.

Your baby will also show a greater capacity for distinguishing different people, different objects, different body parts. She will be developing the ability to move one leg or one arm at will, at the command of her brain.

This is also a good time to start building your child's memory. You can do this as simply as putting a pea under one of three cups and encouraging your baby to tap the cup with the pea, and repeating the process, occasionally moving the pea to a different cup. To keep this game interesting for you, play a classical music tape that you enjoy. Not only will it entertain you, but the Mozart Effect might actually help your child's ability to concentrate as she plays this game and builds her memory.

Fourth Month

By the fourth month some children will have developed sufficiently for more advanced toys, including soft, shaped blocks that can be stacked on top of each other. Most babies go through a stacking phase—hence the age-old popularity of building blocks. But you should expand on this instinct to teach basic lessons about shape, the relations of objects to one another, and that what goes up can come tumbling down (a lot of babies like that part, because they also have a whacking instinct).

By the fourth month, your baby might be sleeping longer at night. You can take advantage of this—not only by catching up on your own sleep, but by using it as a time of *subliminal learning*, stimulating your sleeping baby with classical music tapes, played very softly, in the nursery. Quiet pieces, especially piano pieces that are played *adagio* and that avoid *crescendos*, are recommended. Also recommended are lullaby tapes, especially those that offer lullabies in a foreign language that you might want your child to learn later. Again, you can lay the foundation for future linguistic success *now*.

Fifth Month

The ideas of push, pull, stack, and pull down are now established in your child's mind. It is important at this stage that your child learns the connection between action and reaction, between, for example, the squeeze that releases the squeak in a toy. The early glimmerings of a sense of responsiveness and responsibility can be taught here so that commands are linked to action, so that actions are linked to consequences. All of this is taught through repetition. As you spoon food into your baby's mouth, say the words, "More food," with each spoonful. When your baby refuses to take any more, put the spoon down, swing your hands like a football referee signaling an incomplete pass and repeat several times the phrase: "No more food." Then immediately cap the food and put it away. Repeat this process every mealtime.

It's also a good time to start playing ball, rolling a ball to baby and encouraging her to roll it back, or rolling it just beyond her reach so that she has to move to get it, teaching her spatial relationships, and how to use her body.

Your baby will also be greatly entertained—and can learn a lot—by playing in front of a mirror. Self-esteem derives from self-identification, and is crucial for future learning. That process is another that starts *now*.

Six to Twelve Months

Get your child ready for "the Genesis Test." In the Old Testament, one of Adam's first acts is to give names to all "the birds of the air, and all of the beasts in the field."

Your baby should be equally ready to start learning to attach names to things. Teach your child to point to a dog when you say "dog," a cat when you say "cat," or a blanket when you say "blanket."

True learning begins now. Your child can sit for long periods on her own. She has learned to distinguish much about her environment. You can now, in a limited way, start playing school.

Simple exercises that sharpen your child's mental discrimination are to be encouraged. For example, put a spoon between two forks, and say: "Pick up the spoon." And work at it until she gets it right on command. It's also not too early to start counting objects as you name them.

Your baby will actively want your attention now—and she deserves it. Her sounds will have recognizable parts of words. Work with her to develop them. Sing and talk to her more than ever, but especially by linking names to objects—this will greatly accelerate her learning.

It's also time to start making oversized flash cards to teach her the shapes of letters and numbers—and to learn to discriminate between the two. We've included some starter flash cards in the back of this book.

By this time in your child's life, it's possible to start accelerating the learning curve. A child's mind is eager to absorb knowledge. Though her attention span may fatigue early, it is the things that we learn when we're young—from perhaps the age of eight months through our preschool years—that we are most likely to remember forever. Think of nursery rhymes as one example. You're probably more likely to remember how to sing "Row, row, row your boat" than to remember yesterday's shopping list.

Now is the time to begin laying the groundwork for reading. Virtually any book is worthwhile. Simple books that make it easy to link words and pictures are perfect, but so are more involved books that teach a child to sit and listen as you tell a story. The key is repetition. Your child has an amazing memory, and the more you repeat simple stories to her, the more likely they will be stored in her memory—the words ready to come spilling forth when she begins to talk.

Because she is learning to associate words—both written words (patiently and slowly point them out to her on the printed page) and spoken words—with objects, it is possible to teach your child *moral* lessons as she learns the basics of written and spoken language.

This is not in any way a prescription for teaching your baby with a stern expression on your face, reciting the obviously important—but to a baby largely irrelevant—thou shalt nots of the Old Testament.

But you can use stories to teach your child lessons about how you would like her to behave, how you would like her to treat others, and to teach the early lessons that children most need to learn about sharing and self-restraint.

> Every child is naturally programmed in the womb to come into this world ready to explore, learn, and love.

Just as important is to remember that learning is a great adventure, and needs to be expressed to your child as such. Learning needs to be taught as play, as a joyful experience that brings pleasure, smiles, laughter, recognition, and progress.

But do treat your child as a moral being. Be honest with her. Be forgiving of her mistakes—but correct them. Be consistent. Teach her the values you want her to have. Exemplify them yourself. And again, be calm, patient, and understanding.

Always stop a formal lesson *before* your child gets cranky. Break lessons up with formal play. After, say, five or ten minutes with the flash cards, break for some play with a ball. And remember, too, that your child will benefit from having time for solo play and exploration. But be sure, of course, to keep an eye on your child, especially as she learns to walk—generally around ten to twelve months.

Once she's up and moving around, you'll want to encourage your child to walk, run, and jump—not only because physical activity is good for her, but because physical activity teaches intellectual lessons. It helps your child to explore her world, and teaches her the relations between physical action and material result—for example, jumping on dirt kicks up dust.

Other ideas: What happens when you splash water? (Most children love the water and can start swimming lessons as early as two months, because they have a natural dog-paddle reflex.)

Or what happens when you run through a field of dandelions?

Or what happens when you hurl a twig into a lake?

Active play also stimulates your child to sharpen her senses. This really is a time to stop and smell the roses, and a time to expand your child's sense of creativity. Lying in your backyard, point out the clouds overhead and identify the shapes they make. Take your child out into the twilight and show her the moon and the stars. Instill a sense of the wonder of the universe. From your window, point out to your baby the sights of a rainy day: the water beading on the glass, rebounding off the sidewalk, splashing up from car tires.

Sandboxes are great—and comparatively safe—outdoor learning toys. Not only do most children love the soft, malleable sand, but it can be used in useful, educational construction projects: carving the sand into shapes, diagrams, and buildings, or using toy cars or toy animals to make tracks in the sand, or making sand angels (just like snow angels), or using the sandbox as a location for make-believe tea parties.

Simple, yes, but the lessons for your baby—about nature, about physics, about social interaction, about physical coordination—can be profound.

Reading for Kids Under Three

One way to make reading fun and easier for your child is to focus on books that are told in rhyme, which make them easier to remember. In this, as in many things, the old ways are best. Illustrated books with traditional nursery rhymes make great learning tools. Because they inspire warm and nostalgic feelings about your own childhood, they will help you bond with your baby. This comforting feeling—of a bond that is passed down through the generations—is one of the great benefits of using traditional stories, which, in many cases date back to the Middle Ages. You can even give the stories you select a personal slant by finding traditional stories that come from the traditions of your own heritage—whether that heritage comes from old English nursery rhymes, or Germanic tales from the Vienna woods, or stories of Irish princes and fairies, or Viking explorers, or African folk tales or traditional Chinese or Japanese stories. It is important to help your child place herself in time and geography, to give her an historical foundation so she knows the way things are now is not the way they always were. This will give her another frame of reference outside of that provided by contemporary standards or by her peers.

But that is for the future. For now, remember that learning to read is not to be separated from learning to love. One of the best encouragers of childhood reading is close parent-child contact. As you read, massage your child's feet or simply snuggle together. Make reading a warm and comforting activity for the both of you.

Be relaxed. At this early age, there is much more to reading than memorization or putting words and sounds to pictures—as important as all that is. Remember that your child is a *baby*. Reading for her is also a tactile experience. She will be just as interested in turning the pages as in having them read to her. She will be just as interested in interacting with the pictures—pointing at them, tapping them—as she will be in linking them to words. Indulge her in this. And if she loses interest in a book and crawls away—let her. Either find another book, or play another game, or let her play by herself. While it's important to start teaching your child early, it's also important not to overwhelm your child, not to forget that her childhood is hers—and yours—to enjoy.

As you read, and as your child learns simple words, you will be bombarded with questions—including that early parent frustrater, "Why?" Be patient, and always take time to answer your child's questions. If the relentless questions have obviously become a game in themselves, where no learning is taking place, and the child is merely trying to get your goat—don't protest and don't get angry, merely deflect, by using a question to embark on another story or lead into another game. When a child tries to goad you, never respond in kind, but merely find something else for the two of you to do. Another strategy is to initiate the questions yourself, using a book as a means to explore. Point to pictures that aren't mentioned in the text, for instance, and talk about them. Make reading an active, not just a recitative, game.

Similarly, don't get frustrated if your child takes a book while you're reading and decides to flip ahead. Quickly bring the story up to the picture she likes and go from there. Eventually, you might even want to create your own stories based on favorite pictures in your child's books. You can write your own sequels to her Mother Goose favorites.

And as you write sequels, you can also create plays. Act out the stories you read. Try using phrases in a foreign language, or give the characters in a story different voices, different accents. You can even make reading time special by creating—with simple paste and cardboard—props that you use while you read.

For instance, try reading your child Thomas Babington Macaulay's famous *Lays of Ancient Rome* using your own cardboard cut-out swords and shields. You'll find that your child will find this advanced book of poetry much more engaging this way—and its wonderful rhymes and cadences and paeans to heroism and lessons of history will become part of her young mental furniture.

With props like these, reading time becomes play time, and like play time, it becomes an eagerly expected daily activity. That's a wonderful goal to achieve. Get the reading habit started and then work to expand it, by giving your children books to read in the car, or in church, or wherever. Books are as essential to your baby bag as diapers and wipes.

Keep your baby's books—at least the stout, hard-board books—on a low shelf where she can reach them as an encouragement to have her read on her own. And be sure to take her often to the library and to the book store so that she learns just how wide the universe of books is. Most so-called superstores—like Barnes & Noble and Borders—have large and friendly children's areas with toys, reading benches, and often story times and guest characters. Take advantage of these.

Also take advantage of everyday items around the house. Go to a low shelf in the kitchen or pantry and encourage your child to take down ten or fifteen items and then put them back. As she takes them down, tell her what each item is—spaghetti, pan, etc.—and repeat the identifications as she returns the items to the shelves. Encourage her to repeat the words with you as she manipulates the items. These can even become story times in themselves, as you build a storyline about the items, carefully pointing to them and emphasizing their names throughout.

Homemade flashcards are another good tool. Cut pictures of animals and objects out of magazines and glue them on a card—one item per card. In big, bold letters, write the word for the pictured item. Most kids will love playing an ID flashcard game. The flashcards not only teach a child to match words and objects, but can be used to teach phonetic pronunciation as well.

You can even make flashcards with the words for body parts, put scotch tape on the cards, and play "Pin the word on the mommy." But be prepared to get a few pokes in the eye. Safer perhaps, is "pin the word on the furniture—like "chair," "table," etc.—or "pin the word on things in your room." The principle is infinitely expandable, and for your youngster, it's a fun play activity.

> Learning to read is not to be separated from learning to love.

You can also make flashcards for actions, and play "Simon Says": Simon says "jump" or "touch your belly" or whatever. With actions, you can start building words into phrases. This is also a good time to introduce foreign words and phrases. Teaching your child to count in English and then to count in, say, German, will not confuse her, but give her an appreciation for the sounds that the German language makes, so that they seem less foreign to her, and that will make her more receptive to them later on. By the time your child is three, she should be able to easily distinguish when you ask her to "Count to ten in German" and "Count to ten in English." And you don't have to limit yourself and your child to bilingualism. The more, within reason, the merrier.

While teaching your child words, don't forget to teach her to read *music*, as well. You can increase the effectiveness of the Mozart Effect by playing classical tapes and helping your child follow along by pointing out the notes on the printed score, the mind learning to connect the printed notes of music with actual sounds—a remarkable learning tool that might even give your child a leg up in achieving a higher proficiency in mathematics. And at the same time, you could be encouraging the development of your very own child prodigy—like Mozart himself.

Saving Your Child from a Toxic Culture

As you teach reading, speaking, and music, you'll also have to face one of the biggest problems that all parents face—and that is, the negative cultural influences that start hitting your child as soon as she watches television or that can be brought to her by older friends. The relentless exposure that almost all children have nowadays to bad language, horrific violence, and inappropriate sexual imagery is terribly frightening. What is especially frightening is its ubiquity. If a young father and son sit down to bond watching a football game, chances are they will also, against their will, be exposed to ads for, say, a "Movie of the Week" that includes car crashes, gunshots, and men ripping the clothes off women. What is a father to do in this situation? Or what is a mother to do if she needs a few moments alone, turns on the TV and flips through the stations, only to exposure her child to a kaleidoscope of inappropriate and even harmful images?

Today, even children's movies are likely to have bad language, unnecessary violence, sexual innuendo, and other messages you will likely not want your child to receive.

How can a parent raise a well-adjusted child in a badly adjusted society? Well, one thing to do is simply to dispense with television entirely. More and more parents who take this route find that it greatly increases their family time and helps their children become more creative as they invent their own entertainment. It also has measurably beneficial effects on children's health.

More and more studies show that sedentary children—and they are usually sedentary because they are watching television—can develop the beginnings of heart disease, which can, of course, directly harm the brain by interfering with blood flow. Other studies suggest that children who watch televised violence are more likely to engage in violent or aggressive behavior themselves. There have even been suggestions that televised violence is injecting our children with stress-related diseases, as the violent images trigger a "flight or fight" response that a sedentary child, eyes-glued to the set, keeps harmfully bottled up. Television is also believed to be harmful to a child's future powers of concentration and memory.

But if trashing the television isn't in the cards for your family, do at least try to strictly limit the hours that it is in use and rely on commercial-free public television or commercial-free cable stations for kids where you have more control and don't have to worry about inappropriate ads popping up. You can also use your television mainly or exclusively as an extension of a VCR and play your children educational tapes or classic films, which is how Michael Medved, the film critic, manages his family's television.

Another trick—besides distracting your child, or changing the channel, when harmful images intrude—is to focus your child on making an intellectual game out of your television activities. Many is the young boy, for instance, who got an early jump on his multiplication tables by following football scores or keeping baseball statistics. Even terribly violent shows—like those famous bad boys of children's television, *Mighty Morphin Power Rangers*—can be turned to good effect if your child is exposed to them at a neighbor's house. Find what's good from the experience, and use it. Perhaps the images your child has seen can help her identify colors (the Power Rangers are color-coded) or perhaps some other useful moral can be drawn—even if it's only about good (the Power Rangers) standing up to evil (the monsters they fight).

What is important is not to panic or to express to your child horror at what she's seen (however violent or horrible you think it is), because being too strict and forbidding can encourage rebellion, or, conversely, shut down curiosity, or, more subtly, attach portentous significance to what is essentially unimportant. A good parent is a parent who keeps everything in perspective. Be calm, but also be corrective, and remember that at least you can set a good example.

Though we can't change the world, we can control what happens on our property. When other, perhaps older, children come over to play, do not let them use inappropriate language. Do not let older children turn on the television or watch programs that you disapprove of.

Shielding your child's innocence isn't fruitless or hopeless or overprotective. What it really is, is responsible parenting, and the more the toxic culture is kept away from your child, the more her mind will prosper. The relevant metaphor is weeding. Weeds are everywhere, but if you rip them out and treat your flower beds with constant care you will be rewarded with the biggest blooms. And the biggest blooms in this case are by far the best—a happy, healthy, well-adjusted intelligent child.

FLASHCARDS

The Study of Alphabet and Pictorial Images

A

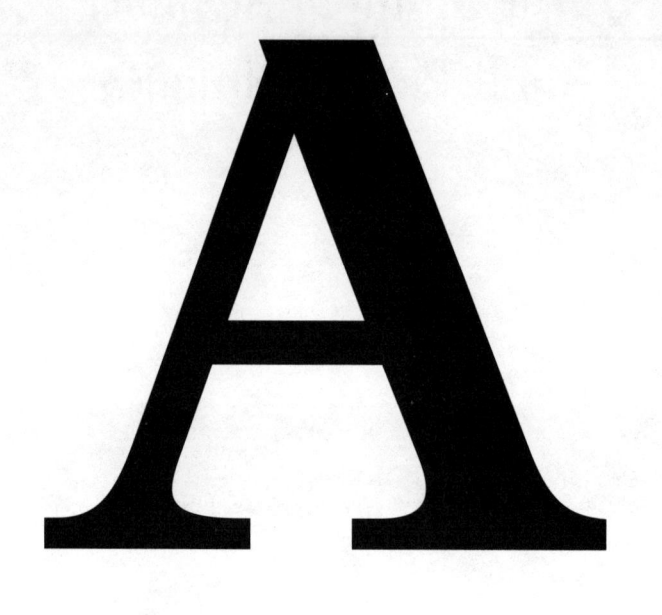

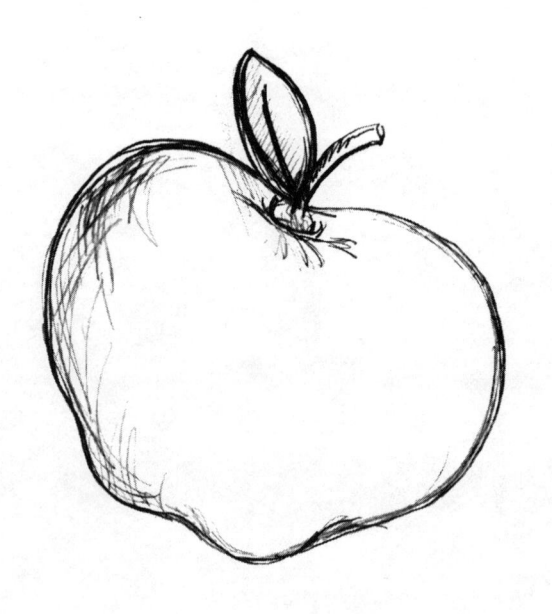

B

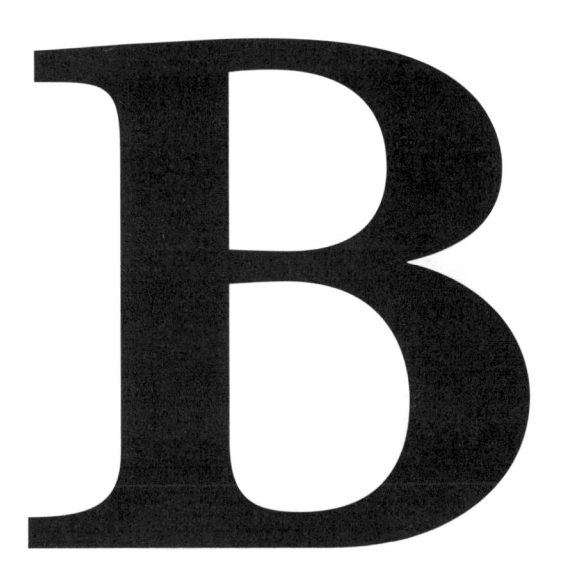

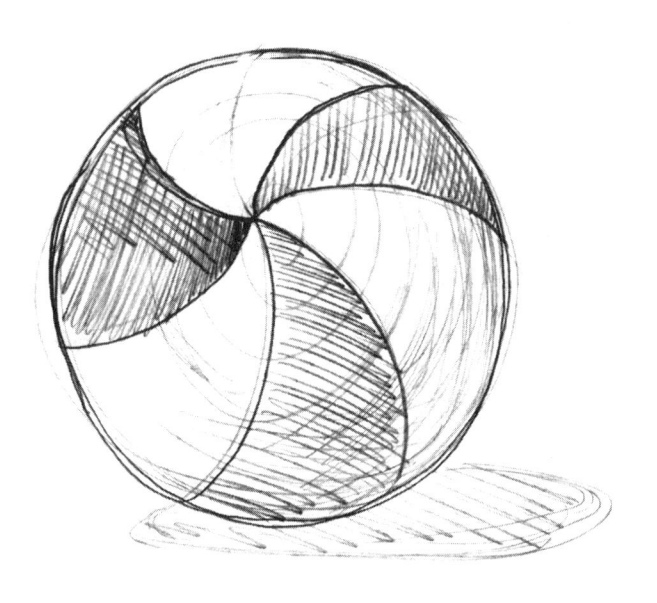

C

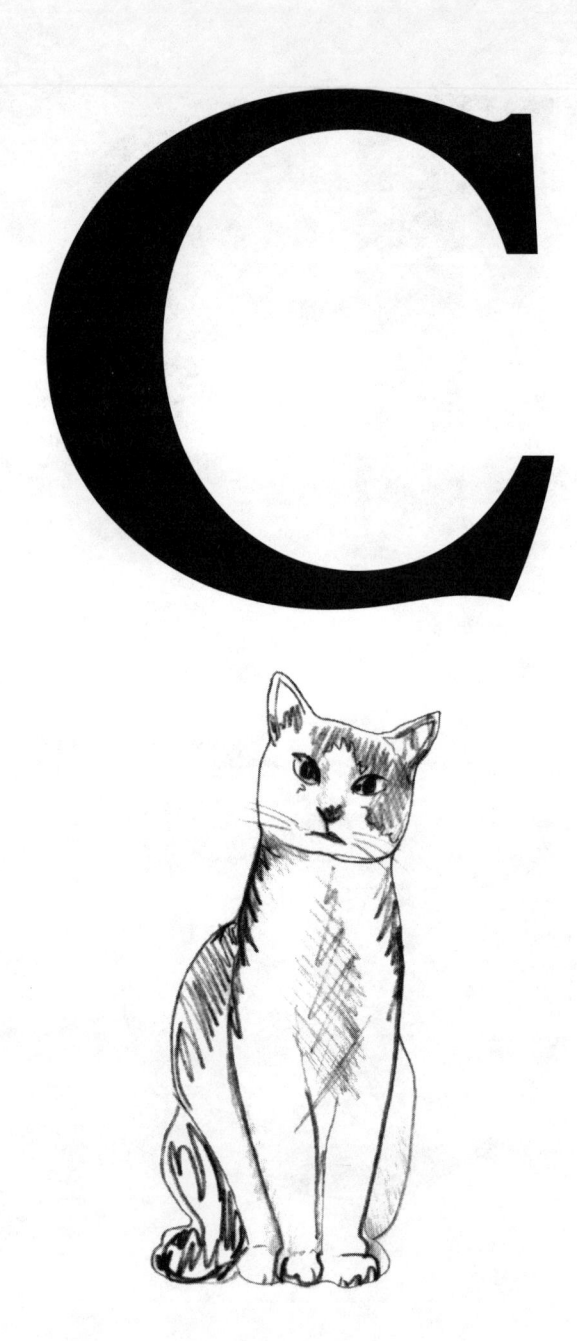

D

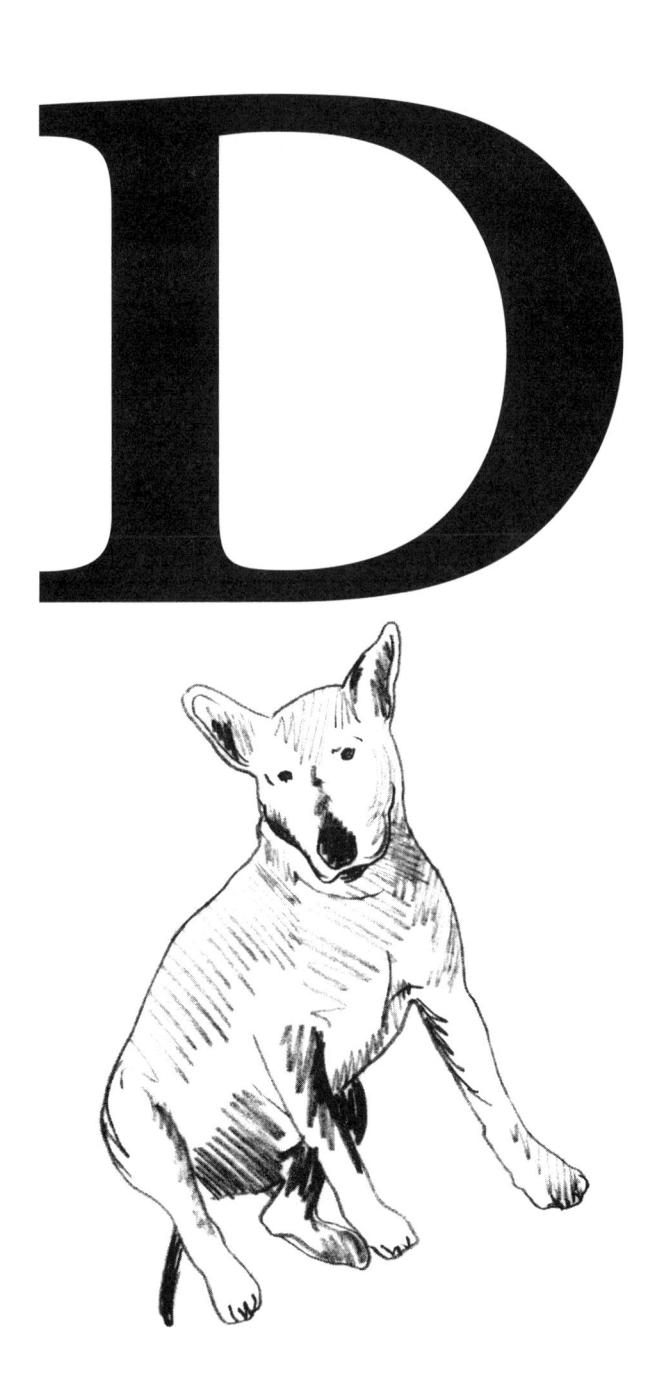

E

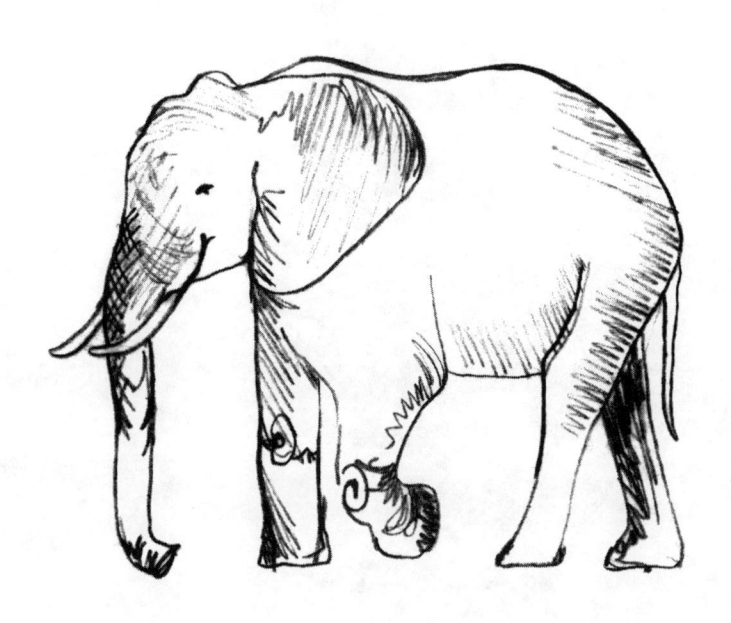

F

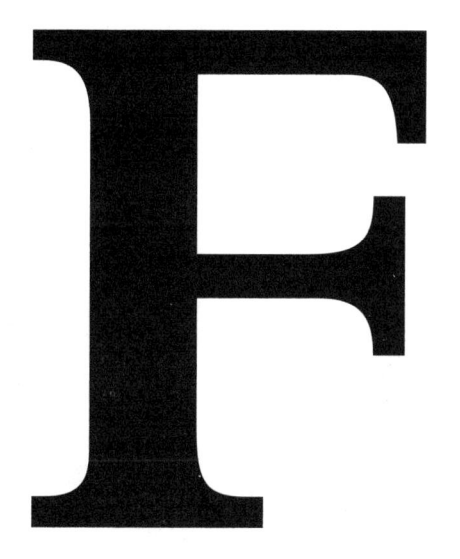

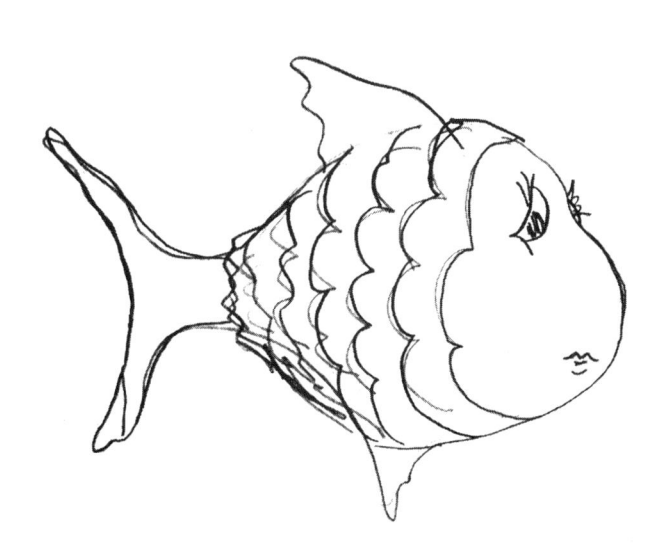

G

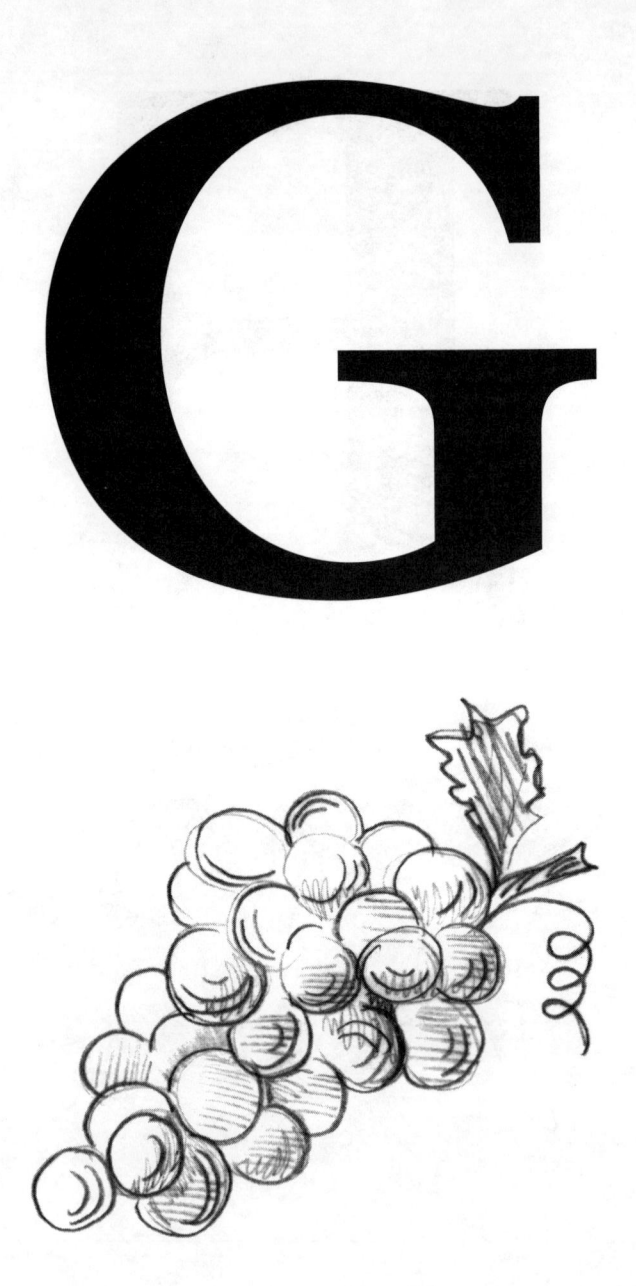

H

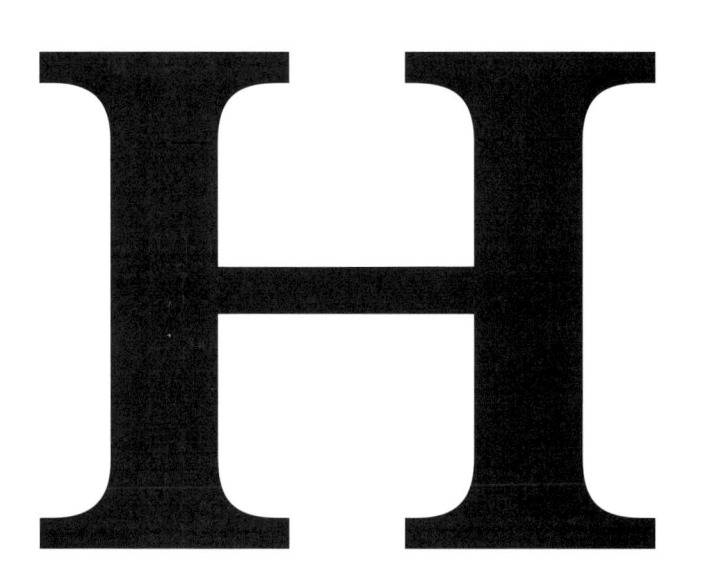

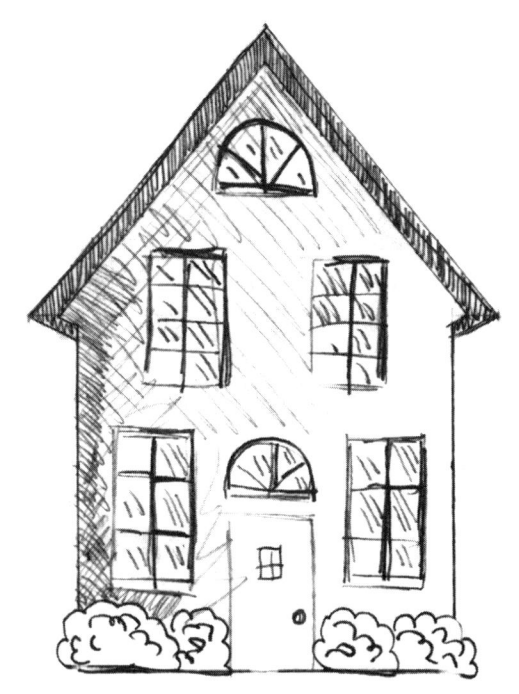

I

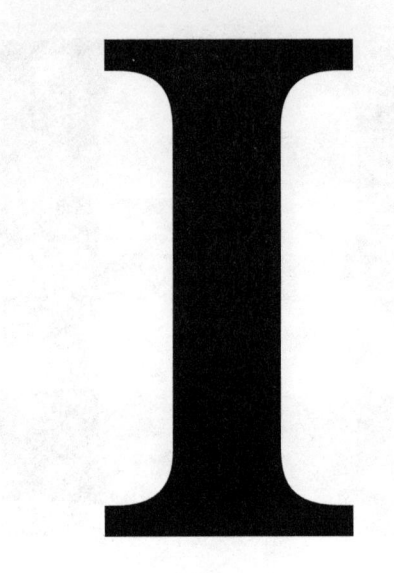

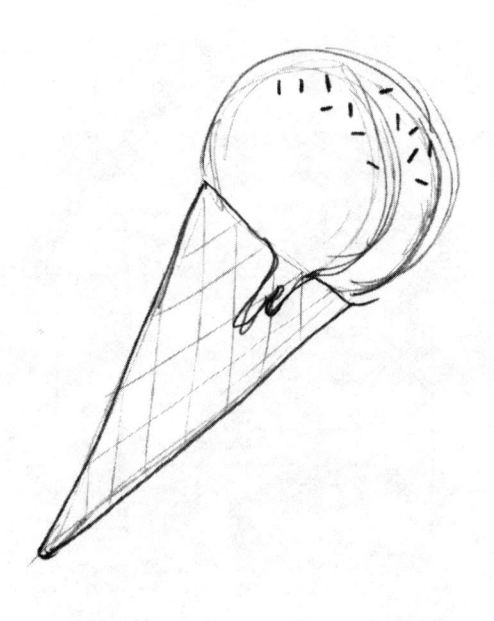

J

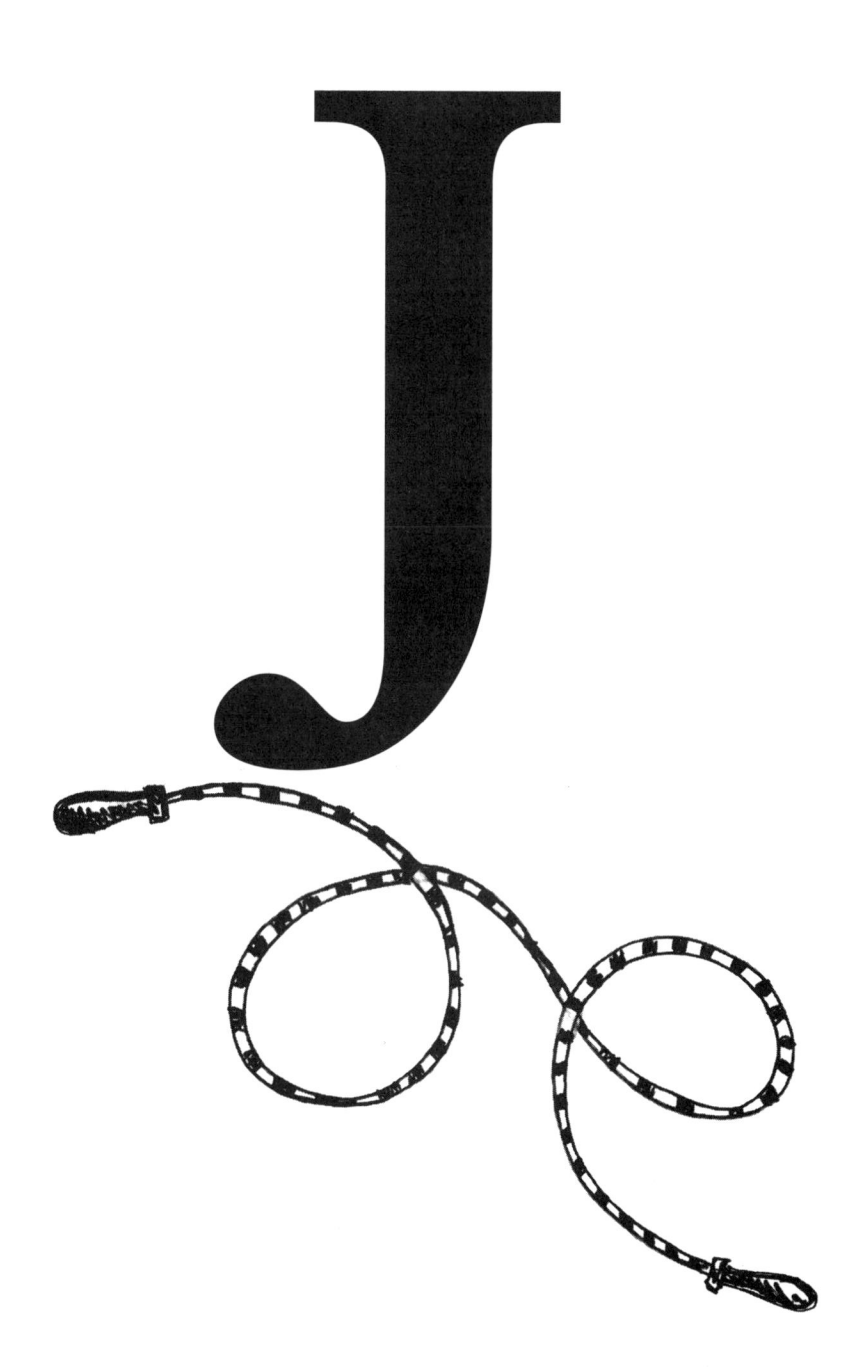

K

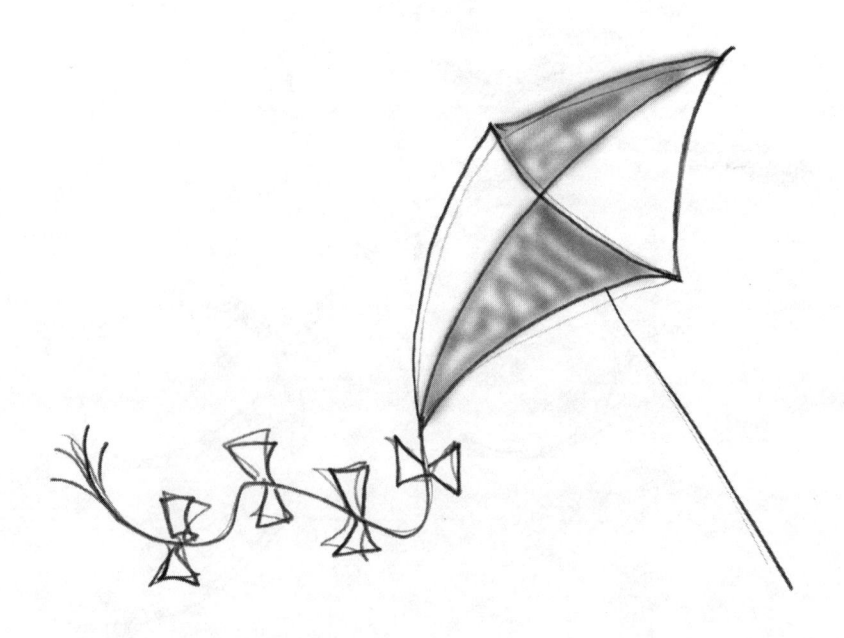

L

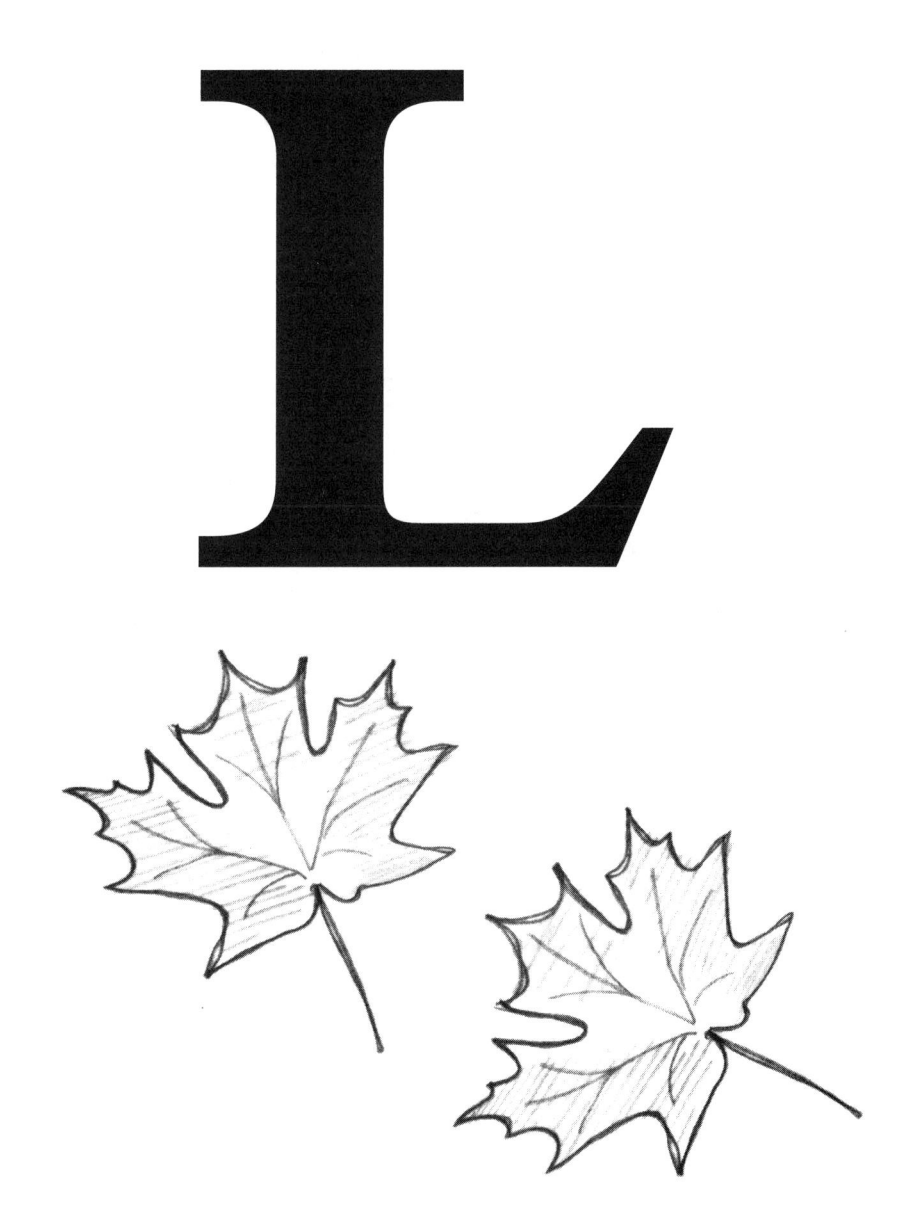

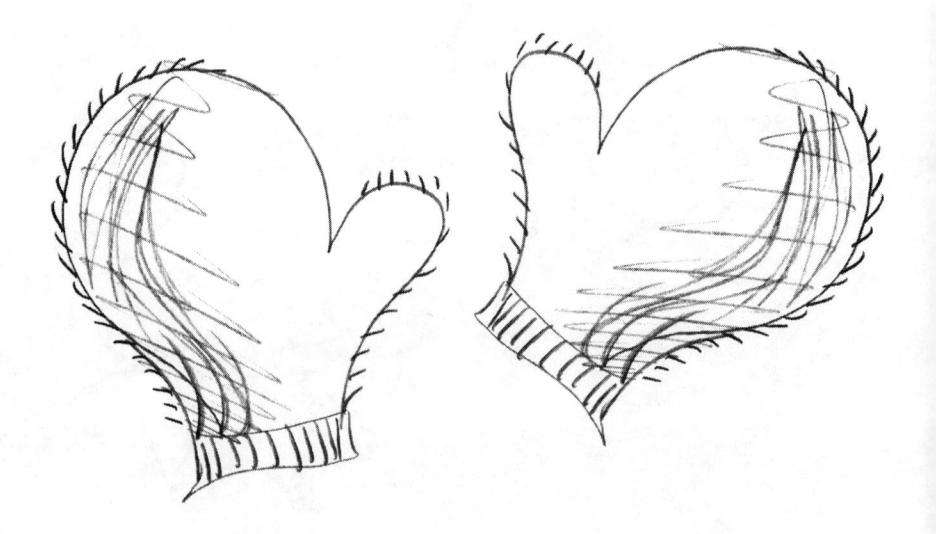

M

N

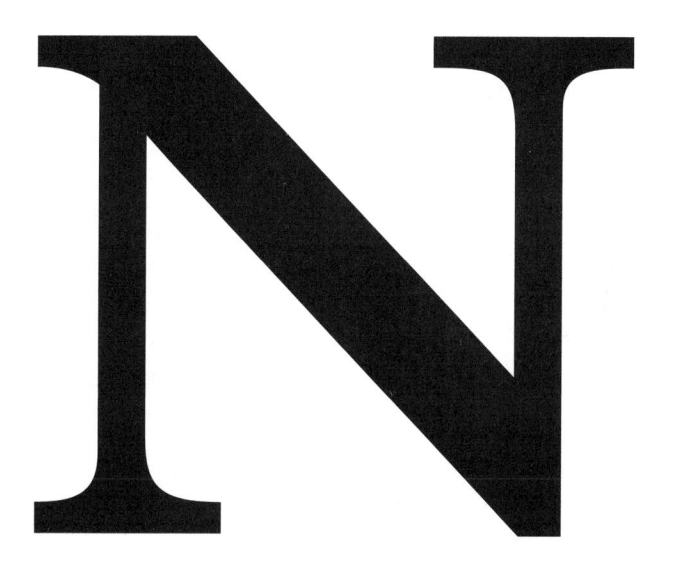

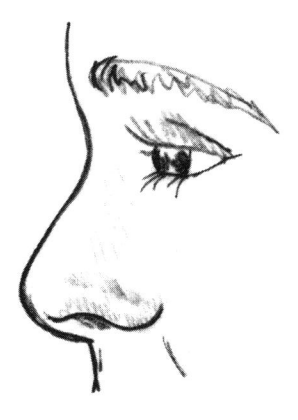

O

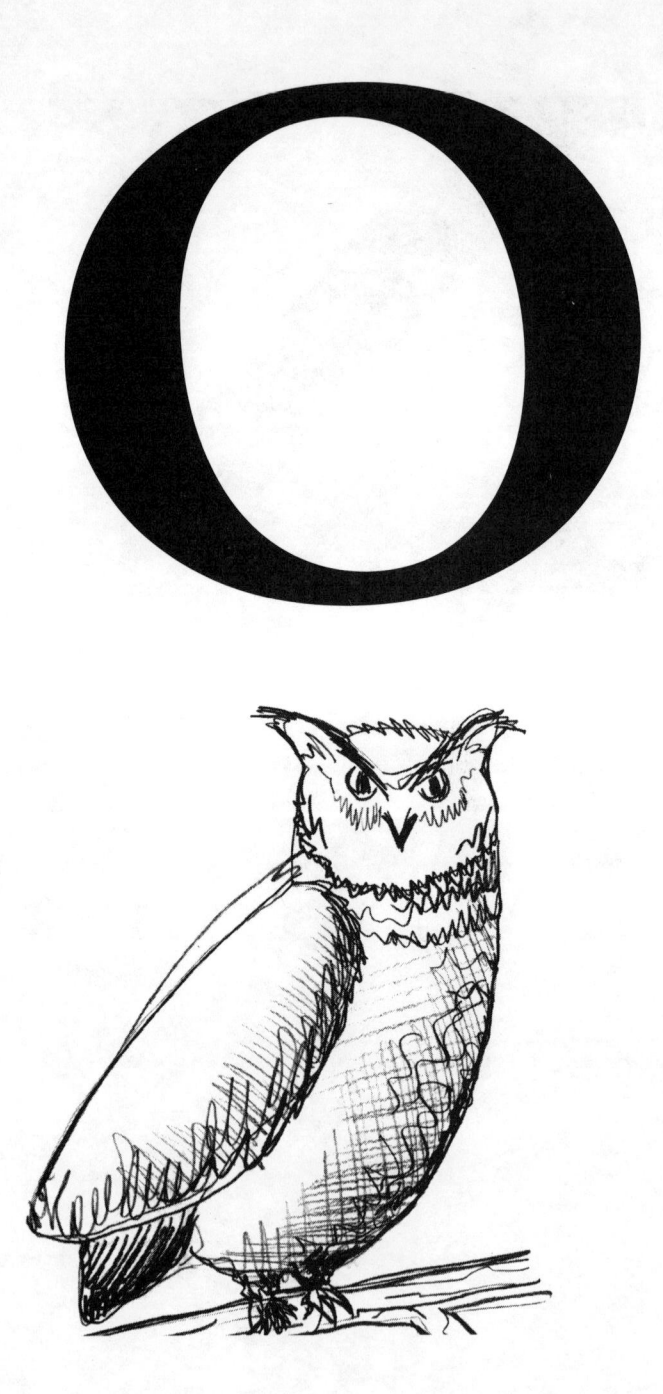

P

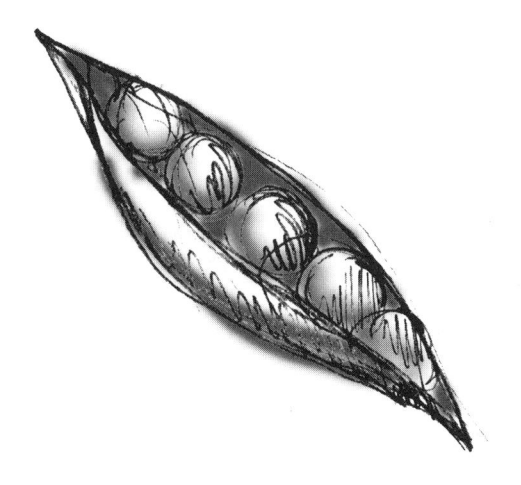

Q

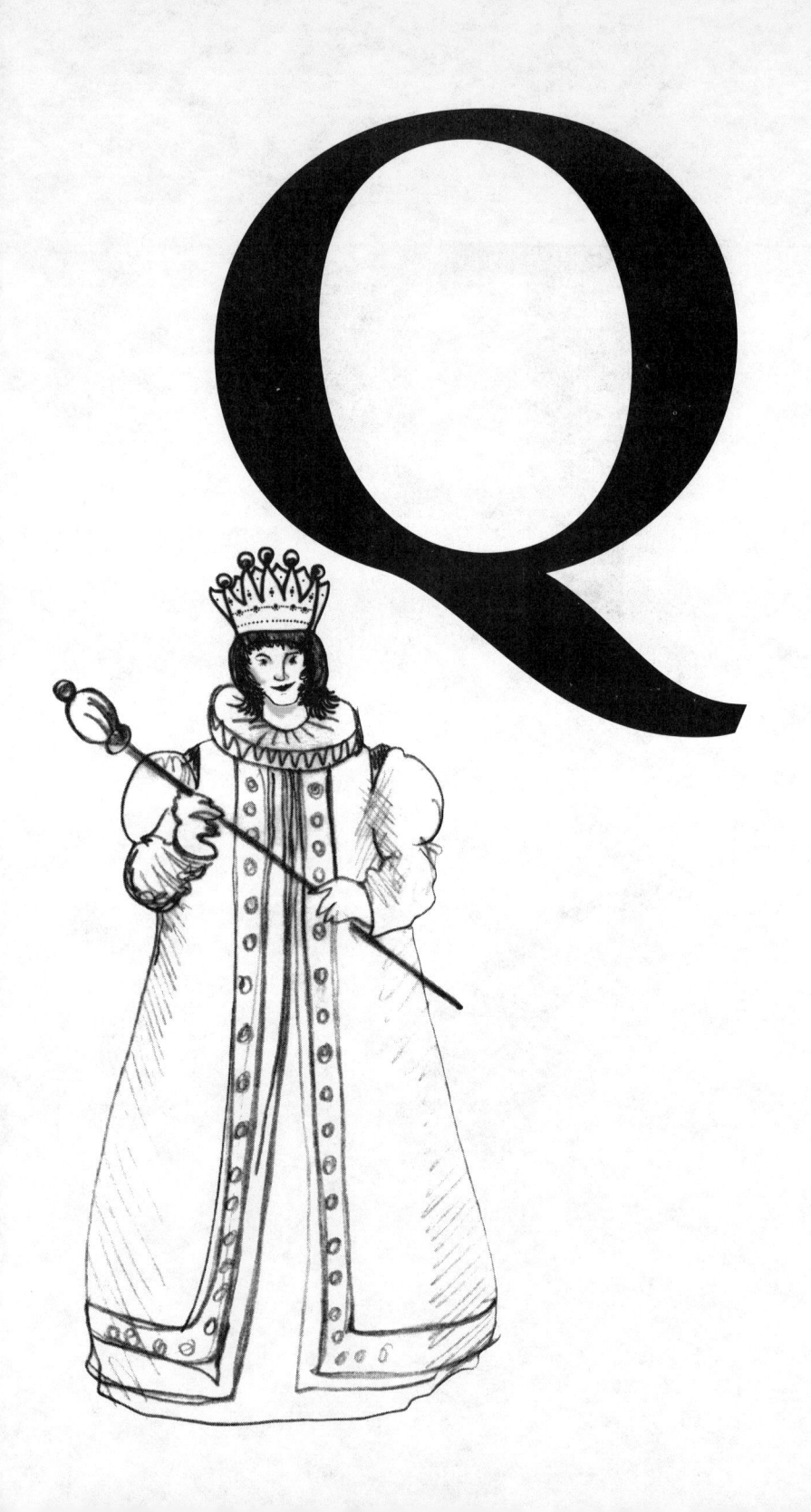

R

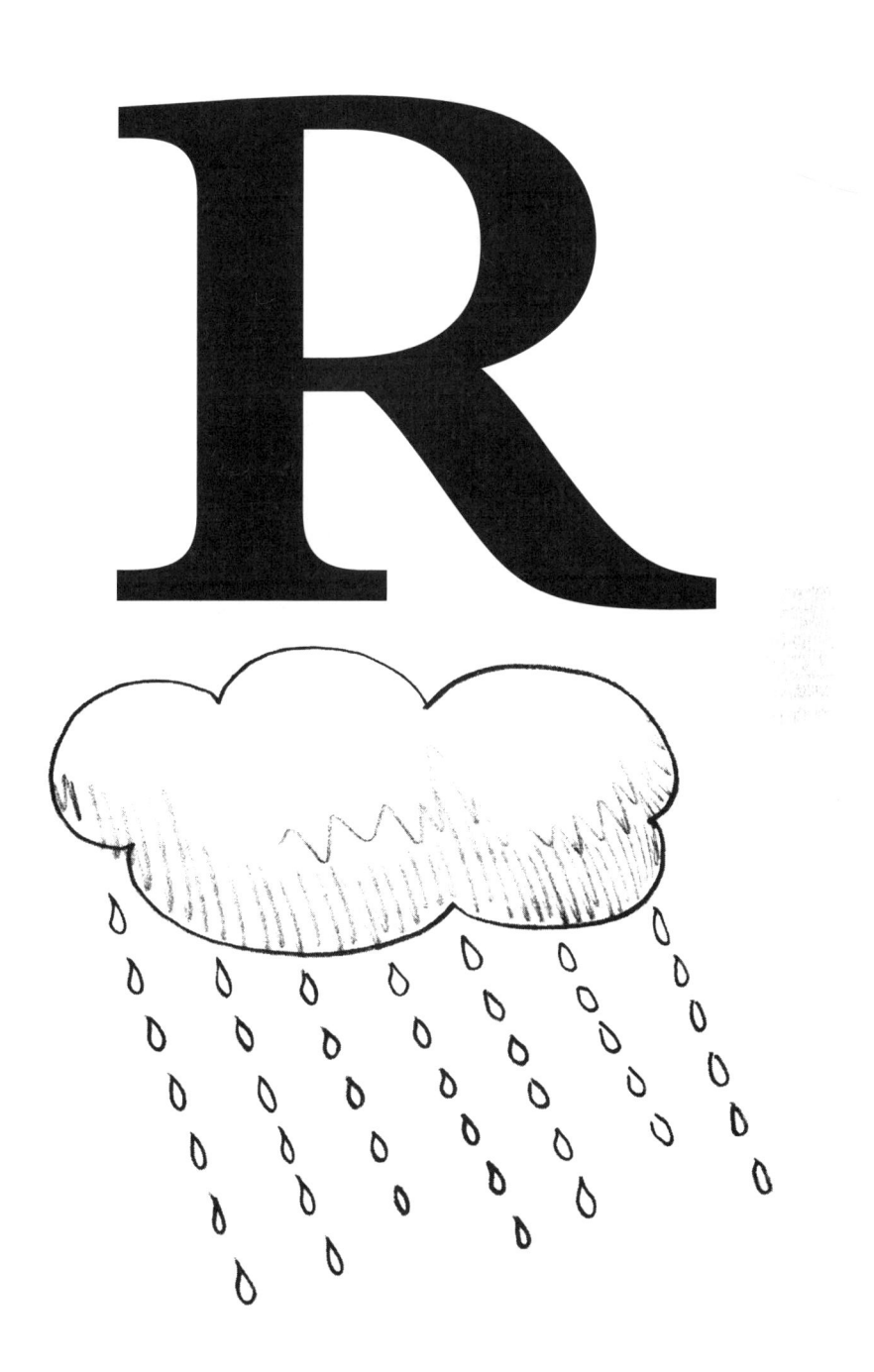

S

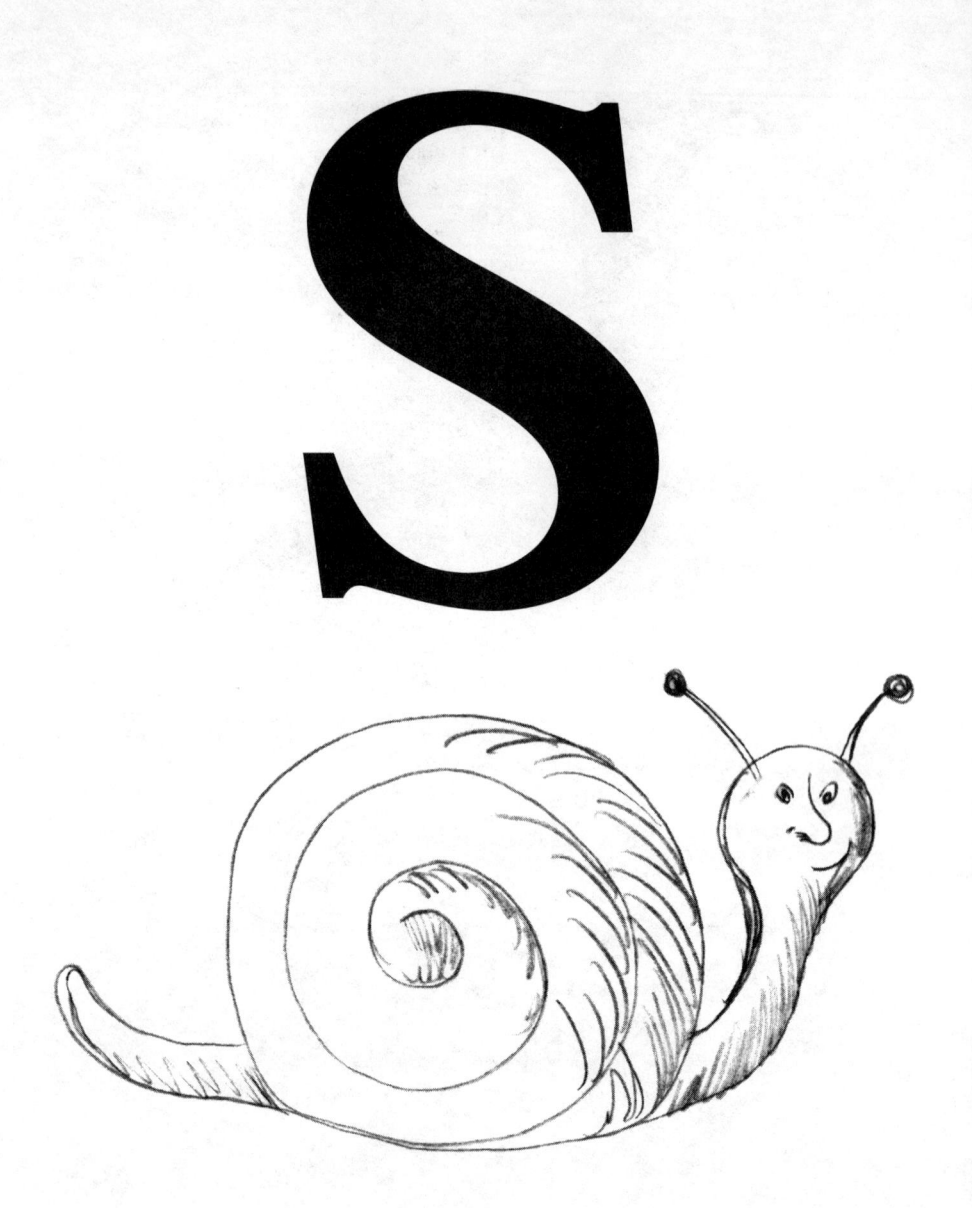

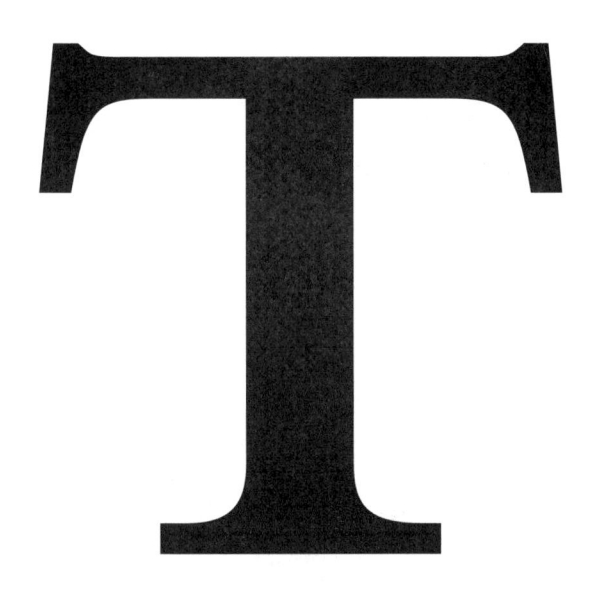

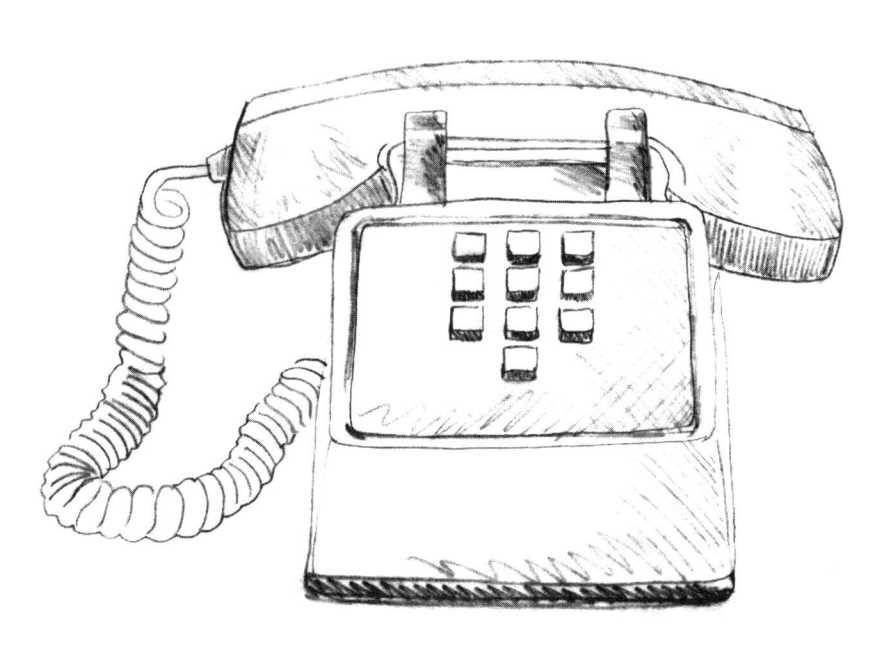

T

U

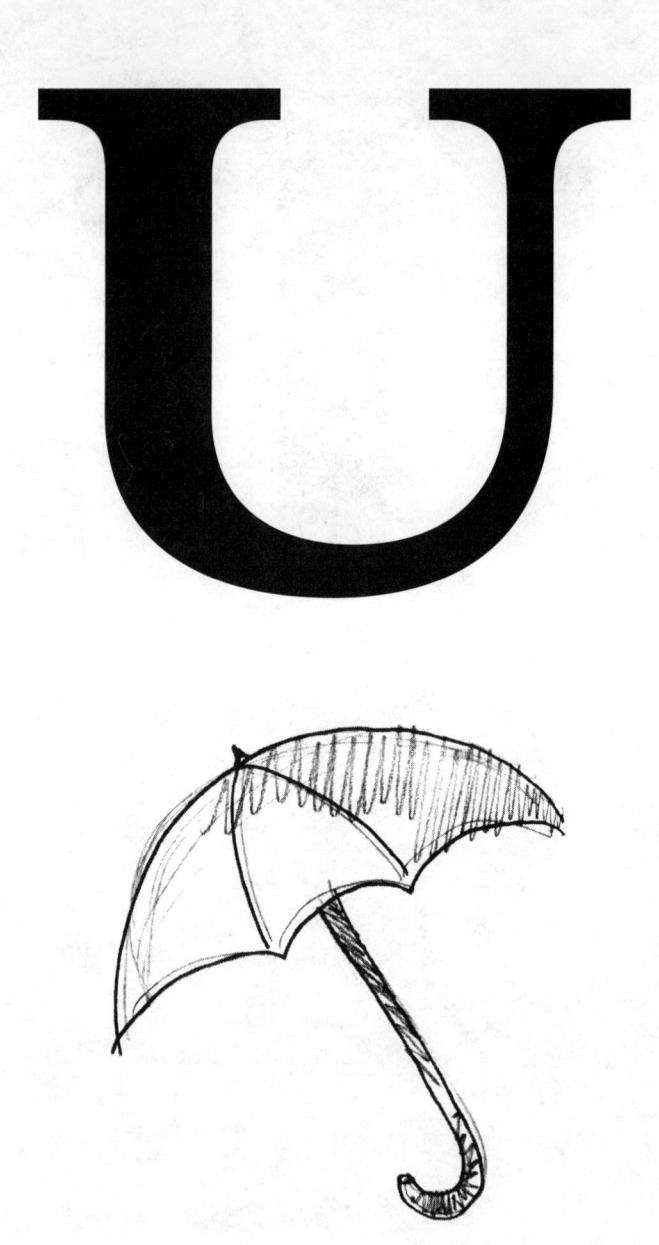

V

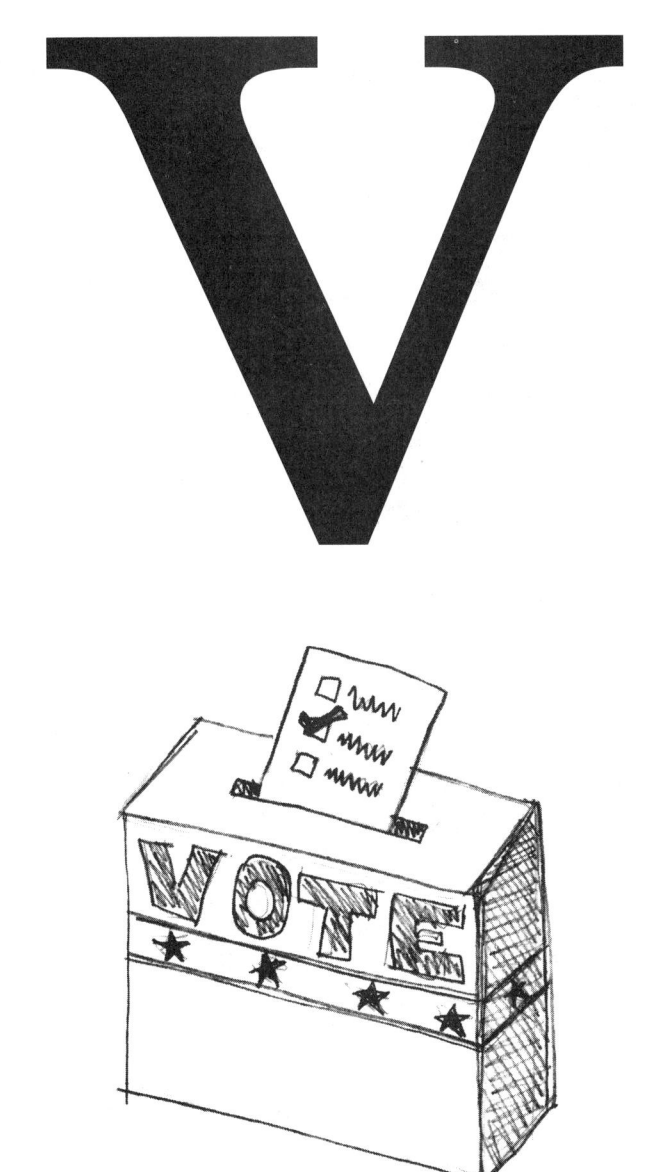

W

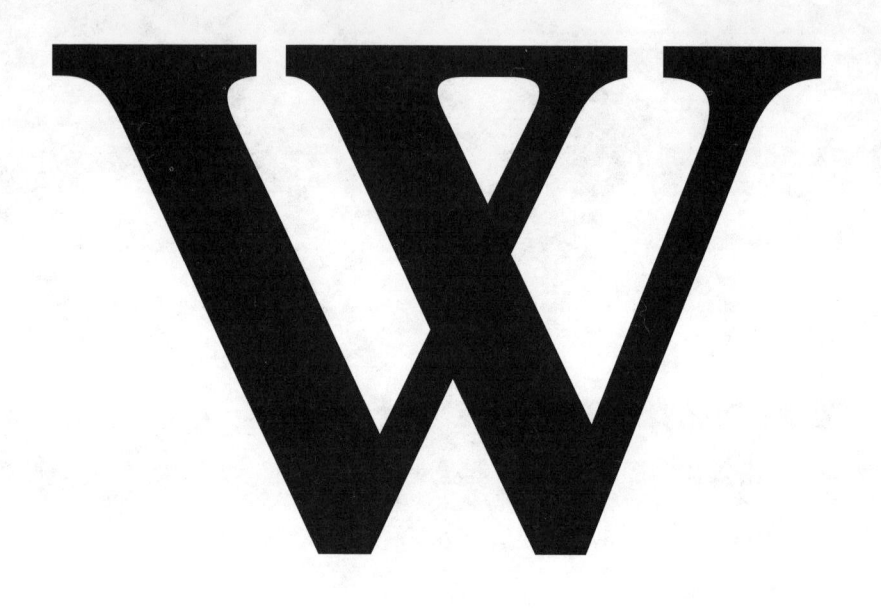

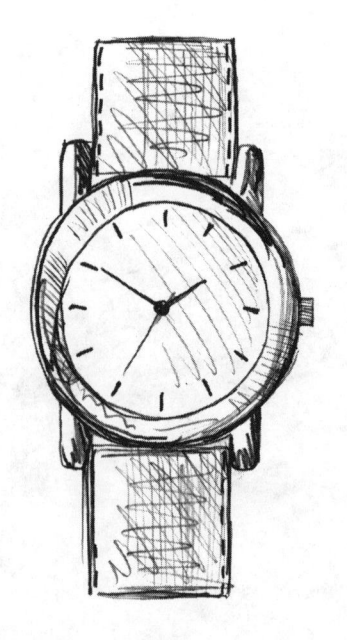

watch

X

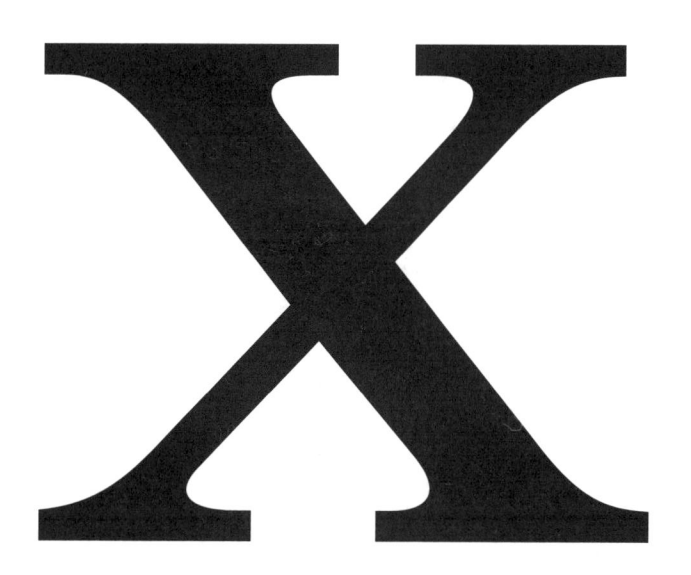

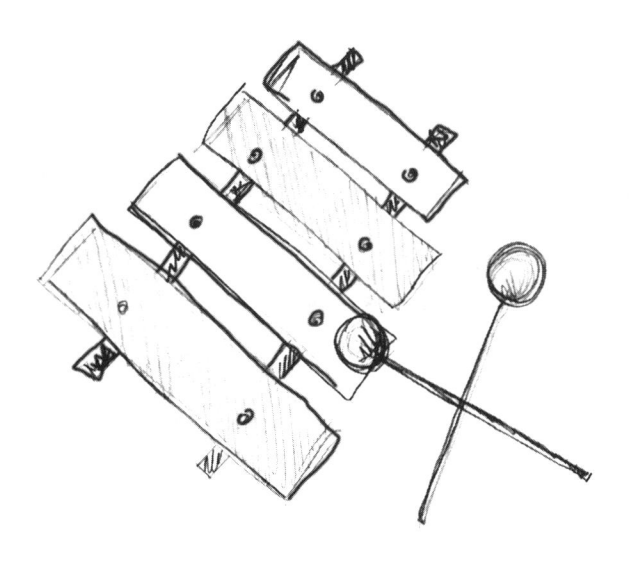

Y

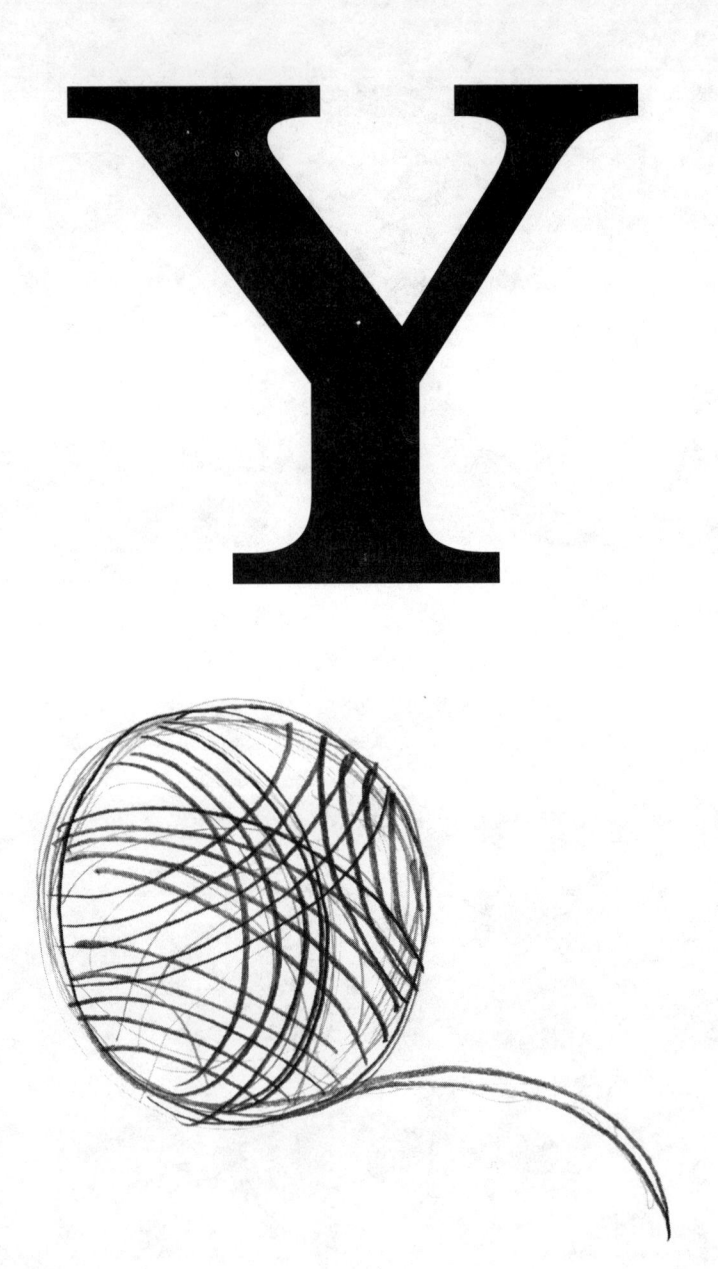

Z

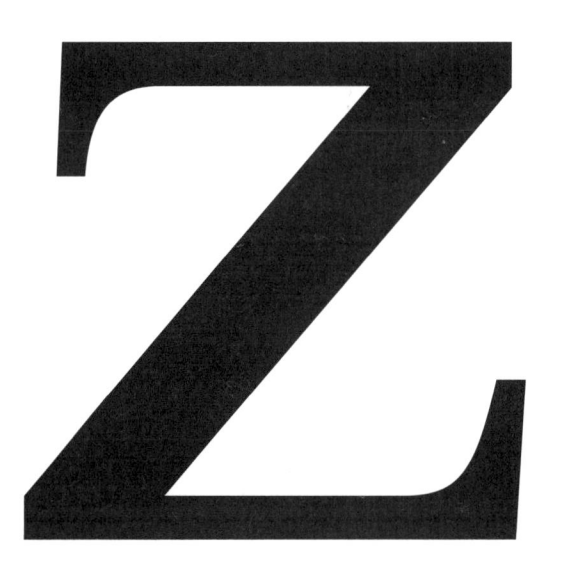

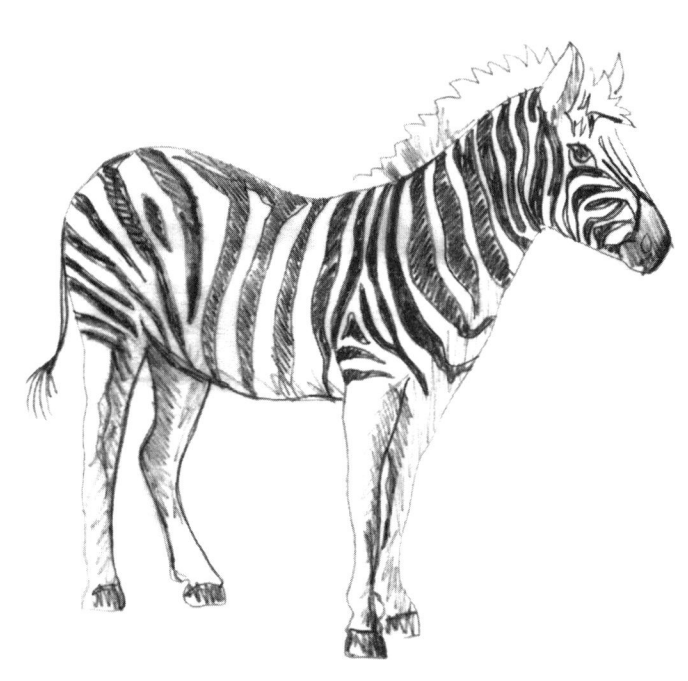

FLASHCARDS

The Study of Numbers and Languages

1

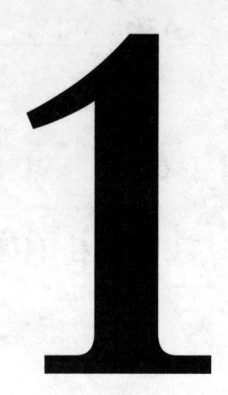

one
ENGLISH

un
FRENCH

eins
GERMAN

uno
SPANISH

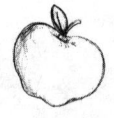

2

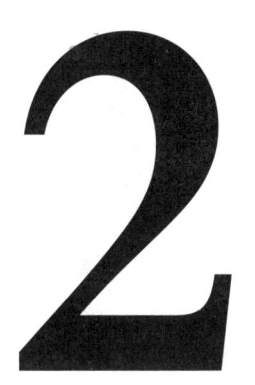

two
ENGLISH

deux
FRENCH

zwei
GERMAN

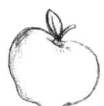

dos
SPANISH

3

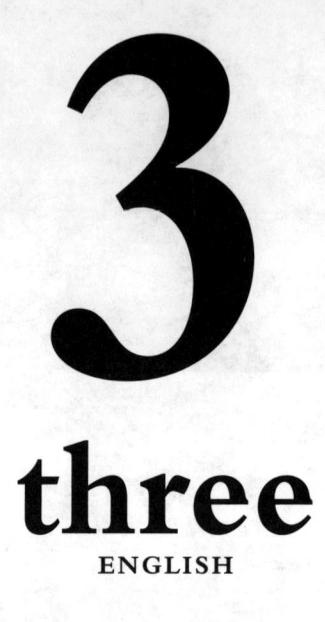

three
ENGLISH

trois
FRENCH

drei
GERMAN

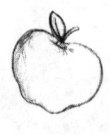

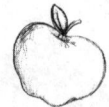

tres
SPANISH

4

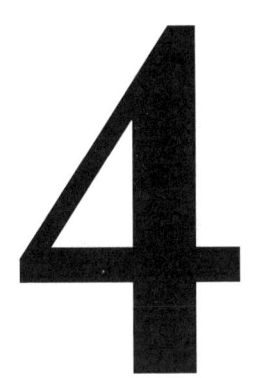

four
ENGLISH

quatre
FRENCH

vier
GERMAN

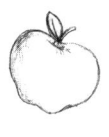

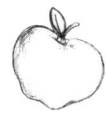

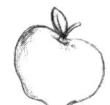

quatro
SPANISH

5

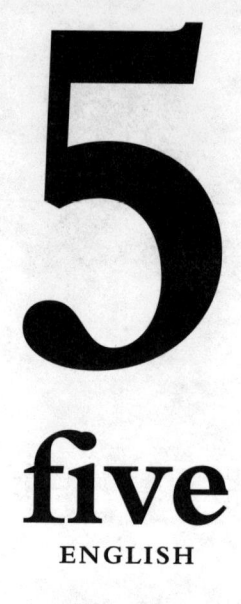

five
ENGLISH

cinq
FRENCH

fünf
GERMAN

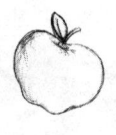

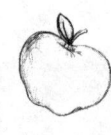

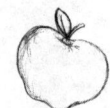

cinco
SPANISH

6

six
ENGLISH

six
FRENCH

sechs
GERMAN

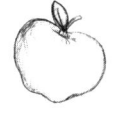

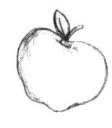

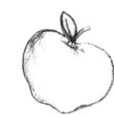

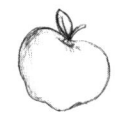

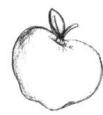

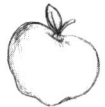

seis
SPANISH

7

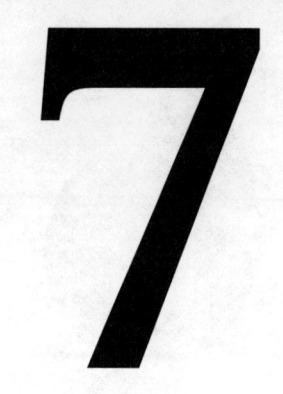

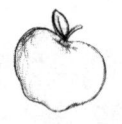

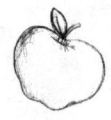

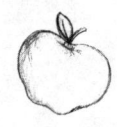

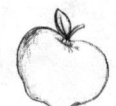

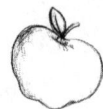

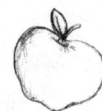

seven
ENGLISH

sept
FRENCH

sieben
GERMAN

siete
SPANISH

8

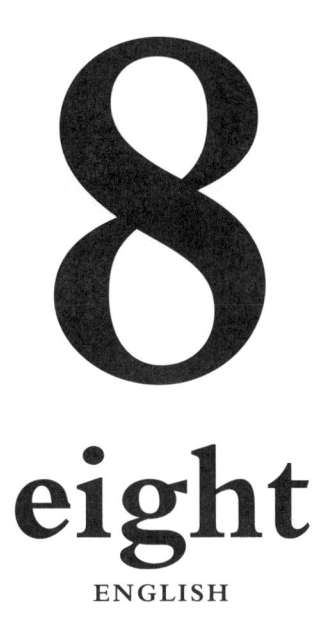

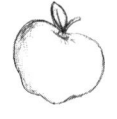

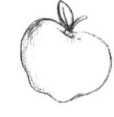

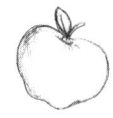

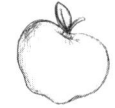

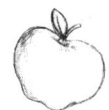

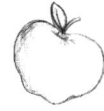

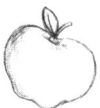

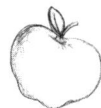

eight
ENGLISH

huit
FRENCH

acht
GERMAN

ocho
SPANISH

9

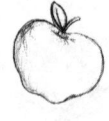

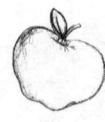

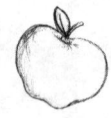

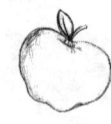

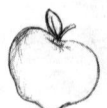

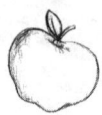

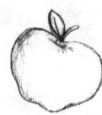

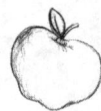

nine
ENGLISH

neuf
FRENCH

neun
GERMAN

nueve
SPANISH

10

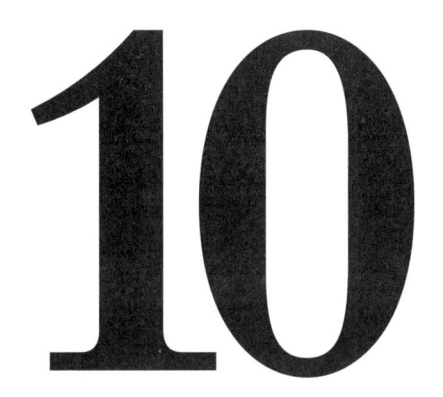

ten
ENGLISH

dix
FRENCH

zehn
GERMAN

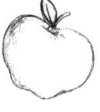

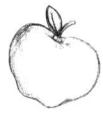

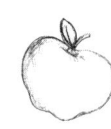

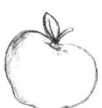

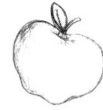

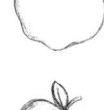

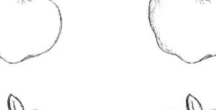

diez
SPANISH

APPENDIX

Intriguing Touch Studies from the Animal Kingdom

Tactile stimulation is universally provided by mammals to their young. So it is not surprising that the studies referred to here show that laboratory animals given even small amounts of extra handling frequently grow up to be superior in various physical and adaptive respects, while those who are deprived of even the basic touch of their mothers are often wounded evermore. Here we present studies involving several different species to show that lack of touch can have a negative impact on an animal's immune system or social behavior, and to reconfirm the research presented earlier that touch enhances and cures. To give just one quick example, as a result of studies linking touch to growth, the Australian Department of Agriculture began a program to knead the backs of baby pigs. The massaged piglets grew 30 percent faster.

It may seem strange or cruel to use animals in research studies where they give them, or deprive them, of various tactile and kinesthetic sensations. In no way do we advocate cruel treatment to animals; we believe it is an unfortunate part of scientific studies. Nevertheless the touch research on animals reported here led to similar observations about the effects of touch on infants and expanded our understanding of the importance of human touch. Animal research led the way for research on the importance of touch and massage for human babies. Although the results of animal studies can be generalized to humans only with caution, there is growing evidence that studies of human deprivation, namely those by Dr. R.A. Spitz and Dr. M.L. Mason, and those on the effects of extra stimulation on newborns presented in earlier chapters confirm the results of animal studies. Stimulus enrichment is beneficial in making stronger, smarter animal *and* human babies.

For Best Results, Touch Your Rats

One of the earliest studies on the effect of touch on animals occurred in the early 1920s and was largely ignored. Anatomist Fredrick Hammett reported that rats that had been taken from their cage and routinely petted by a night lab worker were less apprehensive and high strung than those who had not been handled as much. In fact they better tolerated having surgery. Of the rats who were not handled, 70 percent died within 48 hours of surgery, while only 13 percent of the petted rats died. Other researchers found that handling rats, before weaning resulted in greater weight gain (especially if handled during the first ten days after birth), brain development, and production of more cholesterol and cholinesterase, which indicates brain development. The rats that were petted showed more liveliness, curiosity, and problem-solving ability, while rats prematurely weaned from their mothers showed depressed lymphocyte (white cell) production, and increased respiratory tract infections and premature death. Rat pups that were separated from their mothers did not show distress if provided with adequate physical care and contact and with the specific odor of the lactating mother.

Other researchers have shown brain changes and changes in body chemistry in handled rats giving them a distinct developmental advantage over nonhandled rats. The brains of handled rats were larger, showed more synaptic activity, and had larger adrenal glands. In a study in which handled and nonhandled rats were exposed to stressful stimuli (immobilization, total food and water deprivation), the autopsies of the handled rats showed less cardiovascular and gastrointestinal damage than the nonhandled rats.

When enough evidence had accrued to show that handling rats in infancy had marked effects on their behavior and physiological processes, specifically that they weighed the most, learned the best, and survived the longest, Drs. Victor Denenberg and Arthur Whimbey decided to find out whether handling rats in infancy affected their offspring. From their first day of life through their twentieth, forty-five litters of rats were handled, and a control group of the same number were not handled. When the rats were twenty-one days old they were weaned and the females were bred to a random sample of the laboratory's colony rats.

When the second generation of rats was fifty days old they were weighed and given open field tests. The rats from handled mothers weighed significantly more than those from nonhandled mothers, were more active, and showed less "anxiety" or timidity. Just swaddling rat pups snugly for ten minutes a day during the first two weeks of life results in their engaging in more exploratory behavior. When sound stimulation was added to the swaddling, the pups gained more weight and opened their eyes earlier than either swaddled-only pups or pups receiving neither the swaddling or the stimulation.

Lack of Touch Can Influence Genes

Some studies are beginning to suggest that a lack of touch for animal babies may even alter the activity (or "expression") of genes designed to regulate certain growth processes. Rat pups—taken away from the mother for even a short period of time, switch into a "survival mode" in which energy and water are conserved and behavioral patterns change to those more adapted to survival than to growth. Genes stop sending certain messages. Ornithine decarboxylase (ODC) activity (known to be a sensitive index of tissue growth) stops after only ten to fifteen minutes of separation from the mother. Growth of some parts of the brain and all body organs, including the heart and liver, stops. Production of prolactin and insulin, hormones which promote proper growth, decreases.

The shutdown of these and other processes that occurred during the survival mode were reversed within two hours with tactile stimulation; that is, by using a paintbrush dipped in water to stroke the pups in a way that duplicated the mother's "lick."

Age also made a difference. The tactile stimulation worked completely with eight-day-old rat pups that cannot hear, see, or smell well. For older rat pups that can see and hear, tactile stimulation only partially helps the biochemical responses, suggesting that the effects of the stimulation are specific to the rat's stage of development. Understanding the biochemical and genetic mechanisms underlying growth retardation of rats deprived of their mothers could have significant implications for the human "failure-to-thrive" condition, now referred to as "reactive attachment disorder," and for "psychosocial dwarfism," a retardation of growth and behavioral development in children.

The Value of Nonhuman Primate Research

Nonhuman primate research has resulted in major advances in understanding, among other systems, cardiovascular, reproductive, and visual physiology as well as sensorimotor functions. It has also contributed a great deal of information regarding early social attachment, cognitive development, and the long-term effects of stress or deprivation caused by such human experiences as hospitalization and death.

Touch Therapy

In one study three-month-old "therapist" monkeys were put in with older monkeys that had been reared in isolation to prove that "touch" can heal. Although the older "isolate" monkeys retreated into the corner and rolled up into a ball when the younger monkeys appeared, the youngsters, nevertheless, quickly initiated their normal pattern of physical contact by running over and clinging to the isolates. Soon it was reciprocated by the older monkeys, who gradually began to initiate contact. After four or five months, the effects of isolation on the older monkeys were reversed. In other words, the power of touch can undo the social and psychological harm inflicted by periods of physical isolation, at least up to a point.

This resiliency has also been demonstrated with infant mice, who experienced an initial ten weeks of isolation from other animals. Compared with group-reared mice, the isolates were hyperreactive and displayed either extreme withdrawal or extreme aggressiveness. When the isolates were placed with groups of mice for an additional ten weeks ("group therapy") their behavior matched that of animals that had never been isolated.

Lack of Touch Wounds in Many Ways

Subsequent studies with nonhuman primates in the 1960s, especially those of Dr. Martin Reite, then at the University of Colorado Medical Center, showed that at first baby pigtail macaque monkeys deprived of their mother's touch become agitated and upset. They'd search for their mothers and exhibited the typical distress sound of their species. Their heart rate, body temperature, and serum cortisol also increased.

After a couple of days of separation, the monkeys huddled in corners and had sad facial expressions. Rather than showing stress and agitation, they showed physiological signs of being depressed. Their heart rates and body temperatures decreased; cardiac arrhythmias, or irregular heart beats, increased; and their night sleep patterns changed, with more frequent arousals. Their brain wave patterns showed less REM (rapid eye movement) sleep, and it took them longer to shift into "slow wave" (deep) sleep. Results paralleling that of the monkeys (agitation, depression, temperature, and heart rate changes) have been reported for hospitalized preschool children who were receiving chemotherapy for childhood cancer.

Early social deprivation and lack of maternal touch experiences of rhesus monkeys during the first year of life produces male and female individuals that have grossly abnormal social and sexual behavior. It also results in increased hypersensitivity to the psychotic-like effects of even low doses of d-amphetamine (AMPH) for as long as two to three years later, suggesting that deprivation changes neurochemical systems in the brains of the monkeys. With the administration of AMPH, previously isolated monkeys became hyperaggressive and had higher levels of norepinephrine in their cerebrospinal fluid than did socially reared monkeys. While vulnerability to AMPH-induced psychosis varies widely, high doses can induce a schizophrenia-like, paranoid psychosis in normal humans and low doses can exacerbate the symptoms of some schizophrenic patients. The differential responses of some schizophrenic patients to AMPH could be due to the impact of a disrupted social development.

Lack of Touch Damages the Immune System

Evidence is accumulating to show that maternal deprivation and lack of touch definitely changes immune function in a number of ways. Under certain conditions when lymphocytes should be produced, touch-deprived monkeys showed, instead, decreased production. Studies of young children separated from their mothers by hospitalization for the birth of another child showed the same physiological changes as well as increased illness.

Monkeys raised with each other, without benefit of a mother, also show increased production of certain stress hormones when separated even briefly. In one study researchers noted how separated monkeys, once returned to their mothers, usually perk up again, but some remain forever "wounded"; that is, they are more prone to illness in the future, which is likely related to a damaged immune system. Their heart rate, brain waves, and sleep patterns never quite return to normal, and they have difficulty socializing with other monkeys. These long-term effects get worse the longer the monkeys are isolated from their mothers. Even the short separation (ten to fourteen days) of nine monkeys from their mothers during their first year altered their immunological function into adulthood.

Dr. Stephen J. Suomi and his colleagues monitored the ability of infant rhesus monkeys to produce antibodies in reaction to tetanus injections. The monkeys in Dr. Suomi's study, some 1,400 in all, live on an island in Puerto Rico run by the Caribbean Primate Research Center, which gathers them up once a year to weigh and measure them, and give them a tetanus shot and a tuberculosis test.

Dr. Suomi's research showed that the amount of contact and grooming an infant received during its first six or seven months of life definitely increased its ability to produce antibodies after having received the tetanus injection. The research suggests that mother's touch not only helps us get well, but helps us stay well.

Lack of Touch Affects Coping Behavior

Early separation experiences also result in long-term, persistent changes in patterns of coping. The effects on infant monkeys separated from their mothers for six days was still evident as long as two years later when the monkeys were placed in a strange or new situation.

While monkeys reared in complete social deprivation seem to have the same intellectual development (learning ability) as other monkeys of their species, they do become extremely dependent on familiar settings and intolerant or fearful of novelty. Early social isolation also results in persistent overeating and overdrinking in adult monkeys even years after the isolation is over.

A number of studies have shown that while interventions with previously-isolated monkeys may appear to have "healed" their isolation behavior, when subsequently challenged with socially stressful situations or tasks that required complex social discriminations, these monkeys reverted to inappropriate social behaviors and inadequate problem-solving ability.

While few humans are exposed to the kinds of extreme social deprivation that are created with laboratory animals, the research does point to the lasting impairment that early social isolation may have in modifying certain brain mechanisms, which differ according to the onset and length of isolation. The effects of different conditions of early rearing may be manifested in later life and may explain some aspects of abnormal human behavior.

When they examined maternal "deprivation" experiences with humans, namely hospital admission during preschool years, researchers found that while one admission had no association with psychiatric disorders some years later, the experience of two hospital admissions was associated with an increased risk of subsequent disorder.

Mother's Touch Reduces Stress

In general, studies on monkeys have shown that physical contact with the mother increases certain behavioral responses (such as confidence and social play) and reduces certain endocrine responses of the infant.

When infant rhesus monkeys are denied physical contact with the mother, even though she remains in visual, auditory, and olfactory contact with the infant, all of the infant's exploratory behavior immediately ceases. Although the duration of return contact with the mother may be short compared to the time the infant spends investigating the surrounding environment, the return contact is extremely important in facilitating further exploration.

Compare this behavior into that of a toddler, who will waddle all over a room, occasionally returning to mother for a reassuring touch, only to quickly waddle off again. Apparently this intermittent contact is sufficient to help us as infants begin to make our way in, and establish our own understanding of, the surrounding world. It is the beginning of learning to tolerate separation. It is an important stage in developing our social relationships in the world at large. For it to be successful, mother must be there to reassure us it is safe to move about without suffering any permanent loss.

Effect of Touch on the Health of Other Animals

Psychiatrist James Lynch at the University of Maryland School of Medicine performed a series of experiments using mild electric shock to the legs of dogs and horses. As might be expected, the shock increased their heart rates dramatically. When Dr. Lynch repeated the test, however, while he was petting the animals, their heart rates remained normal.

Siamese kittens who were handled developed the darkened fur of the mature Siamese earlier than nonhandled kittens.

In an article published in the *Massage Therapy Journal*, physical therapist Steven Heinrich talks of a study presented by Dr. Deepak Chopra, a Harvard-trained endocrinologist, in his book *Quantum Healing*. Conducted in 1980 by scientists at Ohio State University, the study examined the metabolism of cholesterol on rabbits fed a diet high in fats and cholesterol. Curiously, one group of rabbits did not show an elevation in cholesterol levels and had 60 percent less blockage of arteries than other rabbits in the study. The researchers found that these rabbits, unlike the other groups of rabbits, had a technician who was not just throwing food to them but was holding, petting, and talking to them for several minutes at each feeding. The interaction apparently changed the "peptides and neuropeptides in their brains and bodies, causing cholesterol to be shunted into a different metabolic pathway that was not harmful to the system."

Positive Touch Care

While Dr. John Lilly's work with dolphins was mainly about their ability to communicate, his work allowed him to make a number of informal observations about them. Their contact with humans showed that the dolphin's skin is exquisitely sensitive to touch, pressure, and the flow of water. For the first two years or more of its life, the mother dolphin feeds, carries, and strokes her new infant while she teaches it "dolphin survival necessities." Dolphins are very touch oriented among themselves, and will lift an unconscious animal to the surface of the water, supporting and stimulating it with various touches until it starts breathing again. Friendship between a human and dolphins begins with a touch. As the dolphins come to trust the human more, they allow that human to touch them in longer and longer strokes, and close contact becomes very welcome.

Michael Fox is a veterinarian who has developed a massage program for cats and dogs based on the strokes of Swedish massage. Dr. Fox became convinced of the "miracle" of massage when, after other methods of treatment failed, he successfully used massage to save the life of one of his research wolves who had become ill with an inflammation of the brain (distemper virus encephalitis). Now Dr. Fox is convinced that pet massage is an essential part of total pet health care and maintenance. It can be especially helpful in keeping the muscles toned for pets that are confined indoors most of the time and in easing the pains of aging and degenerative disorders.

Equine specialist Linda Tellington-Jones has developed a repertoire of a dozen specific strokes, known as the Tellington Touch or T Touch, that have been shown to be effective in healing or calming more than thirty species of animals. In fact, T Touch is revolutionizing the way humans interact with other species.

Tellington-Jones developed her technique with horses as a way of healing their injuries and improving their performance. The heart of the Tellington method is a circular movement of the fingers and hands over the animal's body. As Tellington-Jones refined her method, she developed a variety of different hand positions and a scale of finger pressures from one to nine.

The T Touch is believed to awaken "cellular intelligence" by reorganizing the nervous system and activating neural pathways. Since its inception in 1978, T Touch is now practiced in more than thirty countries and is used by pet owners, animal trainers, veterinarians, zoos, and wildlife rehabilitation programs.

One of Tellington-Jones's first contacts with animals other than horses was in 1985 when she was invited to the San Diego Zoo to work on Louie, a baby orangutan that had an inadequate sucking reflex and was, therefore, considered retarded. Tellington-Jones used TTouch mainly around his mouth and gums, and the infant drained an entire bottle of milk.

Tellington-Jones has used TTouch on dogs with cancer to reduce stress and relieve pain, and has helped rehabilitate a black bear that had been hit by a car in Montana and was suffering from severe neurological damage. She even helped Joyce, a Burmese boa constrictor, heal a chronic respiratory problem. Anecdotal letters in TTouch guidebooks and newsletters describe some incredible successes for animals paralyzed or otherwise thought incurable and even indicate that TTouch also works on humans.

In conclusion, we can safely say that a variety of animal studies provide valuable supporting evidence that touch and massage are beneficial to good health and to proven physical, social, and mental development.

GLOSSARY

Acetylcholine A neurotransmitter that enhances brain function, especially memory and learning.

Antioxidant A substance that inhibits free radicals or oxidative damage. Antioxidants like Vitamins A (from beta-carotene), C, E, and the mineral selenium stabilize cell-damaging, free radical molecules in the brain.

Apnea Periods of time in which infants "forget" to breathe for longer than twenty seconds. It is thought to be one of the major causes of brain damage.

Aromatherapy The science of using fragrant, essential oils extracted from herbs and fruits to improve health and well being.

Attachment (See also **Attachment behavior**) A concept developed by British psychoanalyst John Bowlby that says that infant animals and babies seek to be physically close to another of their own species, the "attachment figure," which is usually the mother. Anxiety grows the longer the attachment figure is away from the infant.

Attachment behavior Behavior that results in a person being in proximity to an "attachment figure (See **Attachment**). Attachment is demonstrated by "attachment behavior," which includes keeping an eye on a nearby attachment figure, crying, cooing, smiling, clinging, and trailing after the mother or other attachment figure. Attachment behavior leads to child care experiences of the adult and to love for both adult and infant.

Autonomic nervous system By brain and nerve connections paralleling those of the central nervous system, this system controls most of the vital functions of the body. It is concerned with reflex control of the heart, glands, and smooth muscle tissue, and aids in respiration, circulation, digestion, and elimination. It is comprised of the sympathetic (thoracolumbar) and parasympathetic (craniosacral) systems. See also **Sympathetic nervous system** and **Parasympathetic nervous system**.

Ayurveda A system of natural healing originating in ancient India that uses meditation, diet, herbs, massage, and fasting as a means to a balanced lifestyle and environment.

Body image A mental representation of one's body and its organs, which initially develops during infancy and childhood in response to actions by caregivers such as caressing, touching, holding, and talking positively about the child's body.

Body organs Structures of the body containing two or more different tissues that combine to perform a specific function. When a number of bodily organs work together, they are called a system (see also **Body systems**).

Body systems A group of bodily organs working together to perform specific bodily functions. The nine different systems comprising the human body are: the skeletal, muscular, nervous, endocrine, circulatory, digestive, excretory, respiratory, and reproductive.

Bonding A complex human psychobiological process for parent-to-infant attachment.

Bradycardia A slower-than-normal heartbeat, usually under eighty beats per minute.

Calorie A unit of heat used to identify the heat/energy producing content of food.

Catecholamine Any of several amines with a catechol nucleus, such as epinephrine, norepinephrine, and dopamine, that occur throughout the body and that can function as hormones or neurotransmitters or both. They play a critical role in the biological response to stress. Catecholamines are synthesized in neuronal cells of the brain, the sympathetic nervous system and the medulla of the adrenal glands, and are derived from the amino acid tyrosine via a series of enzymatic conversions. Outside the brain they regulate blood pressure, heart rate, fat breakdown, and sugar metabolism. As neurotransmitters within the brain, they are involved in the expression of such behaviors as arousal, affect, rage, and motor function.

Circulatory system Divided into two subsystems, the blood and lymph systems, it controls the flow of various fluids throughout the body. By its flow, they take necessary fluids and nutrients to all the cells and remove waste products and tissue secretions. The heart, arteries, veins, and capillaries distribute blood throughout the body. Through the lymph glands, nodes, and tubes, lymphatic fluid, which absorbs waste and excess proteins, is, likewise, distributed. The lymph system also includes the spleen, thymus, tonsils, and adenoids and manufactures lymphocytes, a type of white blood cell that helps fight infections.

Control group A group of persons or animals (often called "subjects") in an experiment that does not receive the procedure being investigated. They serve to show the difference or change between those receiving the procedure and what happens to those who do not. If the research procedure is successful, the control group shows little or no change.

Corticoid Anti-inflammatory hormones, such as cortisone, produced in the body by the adrenal glands, as well as any synthetic compound having a similar activity.

Cortisol A stress-related, anti-inflammatory hormone produced by the adrenal glands and known pharmaceutically as hydrocortisone.

Cytotoxicity The ability of a substance, such as a toxin or an antibody, to have a poisonous (toxic) effect on cells. Certain activities that reduce stress, such as relaxation or massage, can strengthen the immune system by increasing natural killer cells, thereby raising the immune system's ability to "kill" cells associated with certain illnesses such as cancer and the HIV virus.

Dendrites That part of a neuron or nervous system cell that receives impulses for the cell.

Dermis A second or deeper layer of skin below the epidermis, which is a semisolid mixture of fibers, water, and gel. Often called the "true skin," the dermis contains an elastic network of cells that contain nerve endings, blood and lymph vessels, sweat and oil glands, fat cells, and hair follicles.

Digestive system Consisting of the mouth, stomach, intestines, salivary and gastric glands, its function is to receive and break down food so that it can be absorbed by the body for nourishment. The pancreas, liver, and various glands in the stomach and small intestine also help with digestion by discharging enzymes that break down food.

Effleurage A succession of firm, long strokes used in massage. It is applied by passing the palms of the hand (usually the fingertips or the thumbs for children) over a portion of the body and is typically used prior to any other massage movement. Its slow, gentle, and rhythmic movements are particularly soothing and increase blood flow and circulation.

Endocrine system A group of specialized organs and glands that manufacture hormones needed for bodily functions, such as growth, reproduction, and general health.

Epidermis The outermost layer of skin, which consists of an almost solid sheet of cells, and is comprised of three microscopically thin layers. The uppermost layer consists of cells that are almost dead, hence the flaking of the skin. Lower layers push the cells above them closer to the body's surface and/or manufacture the pigment melanin, which gives color to the skin and helps protect it from strong light rays.

Ethology The science of animal behavior, preferably in its natural environment. A basic component of human nature, according to ethologists, is the propensity for the young of a species to make bonds or attachments to particular adult members of that species.

Excretory system Consisting of the large intestines, kidneys, bladder, liver, skin, and lungs, its function is to eliminate the waste products of the body.

Experimental group In research studies, a group of persons who receive the procedure or treatment being investigated. Any changes in the group are compared to a control group that does not receive the same procedure in order to show that the procedure being studied works or is successful.

Flexion What we commonly think of as the fetal position. The baby's arms are bent at the elbow, and legs at the knees.

Full-term baby A baby born between thirty-eight and forty-two weeks of gestation.

Gavage feeding Placing a tube down an infant's throat so it can receive liquid food directly into the stomach. Used for preterm babies whose sucking reflex is too immature for them to take food by mouth.

Gestation Being in the womb.

GLOSSARY

Gestational age The number of weeks a baby has spent in the womb.

Glucocorticoids Any of a group of corticoids, such as hydrocortisone, that are anti-inflammatory and immunosuppressive. They are widely used by doctors to alleviate the symptoms of rheumatoid arthritis.

Hypothalamus A part of the brain that regulates such visceral (internal) functions as temperature, water balance, and pituitary hormones.

Hypothermia Subnormal body temperature, which can be a life-threatening problem for any age person but especially for preterm infants who have not yet developed the ability to regulate their temperatures.

Hypertonicity Excessive muscle tone with increased resistance to passive stretching. It usually occurs as a result of disease, partial or full paralysis, head injuries, or near-drowning experiences.

Hypotonocity Reduced resistance to passive stretch, resulting in the appearance of limp or floppy arms and legs. The condition is often seen in Down's syndrome.

Immunity Freedom from, or resistance to, disease.

Imprinting A rapid perceptual learning process that takes place within a limited period of time ("critical period") soon after the birth of social animals and helps them establish attraction to their own kind. It is a complex process by which the young creature learns to identify the general characteristics of a parent and the other members of its species and can be influenced or modified by many variables including sound and the replacement of the animal parent by a human or other figures.

Incubator A clear, plastic, enclosed warming unit to keep preterm babies warm and help them conserve their heat.

Intubated infant A sick or preterm infant who has difficulty or is unable to breathe without help and so is given oxygen through a hollow tube inserted in the throat.

Isolette A kind of incubator, it is a stationary, quietly humming, clear container, often typically set underneath unchanging bright lights. It has open holes in the sides through which nurses and parents can touch the infant without removing it from the container.

Lactic acid A byproduct of muscular activity produced when insufficient oxygen is present in the muscular tissue to prevent its formation. It is present in tired or sore muscles. By increasing circulation, massage helps remove the lactic acid from muscle tissue.

Massage A formalized or systematic touching of the soft tissues of the body using various movements including rubbing, kneading, pressing, rolling, and tapping. Commonly used to promoting circulation, relax muscles, and relieve pain.

Massage system An orderly or specified combination of massage movements that result in a complete massage.

Masseur Not presently used much, it refers to a male massage practitioner. The preferred term is massage technician or massage therapist.

Masseuse Not presently used much, it refers to a female massage practitioner (see also **Masseur**).

Meridian Invisible routes or channels through which life energy is believed to flow throughout the body. Used in Chinese and Japanese massage techniques.

Muscular system Comprised of voluntary or skeletal muscles (ones we can control) and involuntary muscles (ones we presumably cannot control, although biofeedback research is showing we have more control than previously thought), in general its main function is to contract and cause motion.

Myelin A fatty covering or sheath around each of our nerves that protects the nerve and speeds the transmission of messages or impulses from the brain to the rest of the body.

Neonatologist A physician who specializes in the care, development, and problems of newborn infants.

Neuron The single-cell fundamental unit of the nervous system comprised of a cell body, dendrites that receive impulses for the cell, and an axon that sends nerve impulses to the dendrites of other neurons.

Neuropeptides Molecules composed of two or more amino acids linked together by peptide bonds, which serve in several ways as intercellular messengers in the nervous system. Peptides containing neurons are in every organ and throughout the body. One end of the cells leads into the central nervous system and the other end is located in the skin. When you manipulate the skin, you release peptides, which affect the brain. Some have suggested that the implications of this are that consciousness can no longer be thought to reside in the brain, but rather throughout the entire body.

Nervous system That system of the body that controls and coordinates all the other bodily systems. It is divided into the **central nervous system** consisting of the spinal cord and the brain, and the **peripheral nervous system**, made up of nerves. The peripheral system is further subdivided into the **voluntary** (spinal and cranial nerves) and **involuntary or autonomic** branches, responsible for such functions as digestion and respiration.

Nissl bodies Large granular protein bodies in nerve cells, which can be stained with basic dyes for microscopic examination of the cell.

Parasympathetic nervous system A branch of the autonomic nervous system, it helps us recover, repair, and maintain the body, and is activated by relaxation. It increases blood flow to the gastrointestinal system and helps restore the body's cellular processes. Once believed to be unable to be controlled consciously, biofeedback studies have shown that we now have more control over the parasympathetic system than originally thought.

Percussion Quick, striking massage movements that are especially effective in stimulating the chest, back, and shoulders. They include such movements as tapping with the tips of the fingers (used on the face and more sensitive areas), hacking with the edges of the hand, and cupping with the cupped part of the hand.

Peristalsis Waves of constriction in the intestines or esophagus that force their contents onward.

Postconceptional age Used for preterm babies, it is the total of the number of weeks a baby has spent in the womb plus the number of weeks out of the womb.

Premature (or **preterm** or **preemie**) **baby** Any baby born before 38 weeks' gestation.

Progressive muscle relaxation A common relaxation and stress reduction technique designed by Chicago psychiatrist Edmund Jacobsen. Most current forms use a brief, modified approach to Jacobsen's original technique, which employs the sequential tightening and relaxing of voluntary muscle groups of the body in one session, beginning with the feet and moving upward.

Prone position A massage position where the baby lies on his stomach. It is essential for back strokes.

Respirator (also **ventilator**) A machine that helps infants breath.

Respiratory system That part of the body consisting of the mouth, nose, larynx, trachea, bronchial tubes, and lungs. It serves to provide oxygen to the bloodstream and to remove wastes in the form of carbon dioxide.

Reproductive system Consisting of the sexual organs, the ovaries in the female, and the testes in the male, the function of this system is to ensure continuation of the species by reproduction.

Skeletal system Consisting of the more than two hundred bones of the body, its main function is body support for the other systems. It is the physical foundation of the body. The bones also protect some of the body's most delicate organs and assist in movement, acting as levers at the joints or points of connection between them.

Skin The outer covering of the body and its largest organ. It is composed of two clearly defined divisions: the **epidermis**, or outermost layer, and the **dermis**, the deeper layer or true skin. The skin's function is to protect internal organs from injury, and, in general, to protect the body from bacterial infection. It also regulates the temperature of the body and excretes some waste matter through the sweat glands (perspiration). The sebaceous (oil) glands produce and release the lubricant sebum, which coats the surface of the skin and helps the body to maintain its moisture level. On a small scale the skin breathes through its pores and assists respiration. Through its rich supply of nerve endings or receptors, the skin provides us with information about the environment.

Subcutaneous tissue A continuation or deeper layer of the dermis comprised largely of fatty (adipose) tissue. It serves to protect upper skin layers, provide a reservoir of fuel and energy, and give general shape and smoothness to the body.

Supine position The preferred position for pediatric massage because it gives the best opportunity for eye contact and interaction, since the baby lies on her back and can see the caregiver's face. All parts of the body, except the back (see **Prone position**) can be massaged in this position.

Sympathetic nervous system A subbranch of the autonomic nervous system, the sympathetic nervous system is the body's arousal system and is activated during stress or preparing for "fight or flight." It prepares the body for emergency activity and maximal physical performance by increasing heart rate and blood pressure, elevating blood sugar, and directing blood flow to the skeletal muscles.

Tachycardia Rapid heartbeat consisting of 180 or more beats per minute.

Vagus nerves The tenth pair of cranial nerves that extend from the brain down the spinal column. One of their functions is to promote sensations and movement in the intestines and other abdominal organs.

Ventilator (See **Respirator**).

Weaning Withdrawal from breastfeeding.

REFERENCES

Auckett, A. D. *Baby Massage. Parent-Child Bonding Through Touch.* N.Y.: Newmarket Press, 1989.

Almli, C. R. and S. Lofsness. "Preterm Human Infants: Heart Rate and Movement Changes in Response to Tactile Stimulation." *Society for Neuroscience Abstract*, 1985.

Babson, S. G., M. L. Pernoll, and G. I. Benda. *Diagnosis and Management of the Fetus and Neonate at Risk.* St. Louis: Mosby, 1980.

Barglow, P. D. "Prematurity and Infant Stimulation: A Review of Research." *Child Psychiatry and Human Development*, 1980.

Barnard, K. A. "The Effect of Stimulation on the Duration and Amount of Sleep and Wakefulness in the Premature Infant." Unpublished Doctoral Dissertation from the University of Washington, 1972.

Beck, M. *The Theory and Practice of Therapeutic Massage.* Albany, N.Y.: Milady Publishing Co., 1988.

Benjamin, P. J. "More Alike than Different." *Massage Therapy Journal*, 1988.

Bennett, William J., ed. *The Book of Virtues.* New York: Simon & Schuster, 1993.

Bennett, William J., ed. *The Children's Book of Virtues.* New York: Simon & Schuster, 1995.

Bennett, William J., ed. *The Children Book of Virtues Audio Treasury.* New York: Simon & Schuster, 1997.

Bloom, Allan. *The Closing of the American Mind.* New York: Simon and Schuster, 1987.

Campbell, Don. *The Mozart Effect.* New York: Avon Books, 1997.

Ching, M. "The Use of Touch in Nursing Practice." *The Australian Journal of Advanced Nursing*, 1995.

Cohen, S. S. *The Magic of Touch.* New York: Harper & Row Publishers, 1987.

Cottingham, J. T. *Healing Through Touch*. Boulder, Colorado: Rolf Institute, 1985.

Crelin, E. S. "Development of the Lower Respiratory System." *Clinical Symposia*, 1975.

Edelman, A. M., H. C. Kraemer, and A. F. Korner. "Effects of Compensatory Movement Stimulation on the Sleep-Awake Behaviors of Preterm Infants." *Journal of the American Academy of Child Psychiatry*, 1982.

Elmer, E. and G. S. Gregg. "Developmental Characteristics of Abused Children." *Pediatrics*, 1967.

Field, T., N. Grizzle, F. Scafidi, S. Abrams, S. Richardson, C. Kuhy, and S. Schanberg. "Massage Therapy for Infants of Depressed Mothers." *Infant Behavior and Development*, 1996.

Field, T. "Infant Massage Therapy." *Touch in Early Development*, Mahwah, N.J.: Lawrence Erlbaum Associates, 1995.

Field, T. "Massage Therapy for Infants and Children." *Developmental and Behavioral Pediatrics*, 1995.

Field, T., T. Kilmer, and I. Burman. "Preschool Children's Sleep and Wake Behavior Improve After Massage Therapy." Unpublished research study from the Touch Research Institute.

Gottfried, A. W. "Touch as an Organizer for Learning and Development." *The Many Facets of Touch*, C. C. Brown, ed. (Johnson and Johnson Pediatric Round Table). N.Y.: Elsevier, 1984.

Hausner, Lee, Ph.D. and Scholsberg, Jeremy, *Teaching Your Child Concentration*. Washington DC: LifeLine Press, 1998.

Hausner, Lee, Ph.D. and Jeremy Scholsberg. *Teaching Your Child Creativity*. Washington DC: LifeLine Press, 1998.

Jay, S. S. "The Effects of Gentle Human Touch on Mechanically Ventilated Very-Short-Gestation Infants." *Maternal-Child Nursing Journal*, Monograph 12, 1982.

Klaus, M. H. and A. A. Farnaroff. *Care of the High-Risk Neonate*. Philadelphia: W. B. Saunders Co., 1973.

REFERENCES

Kotulak, Ronald, "Gordon L. Shaw; Physicist, Discover of 'Mozart Effect'." *Chicago Tribune*, May 24, 1998.

Korner, A. F. "Maternal Deprivation: Compensatory Stimulation for the Prematurely Born Infant." *Maternal Influences and Early Behavior*, R. W. Bell and W. P. Smotherman, eds. N.Y.: SP Medical and Scientific Books, 1980.

Leboyer, F. *Birth Without Violence*. N.Y.: Alfred A. Knopf, Inc., 1976.

Leifer, A. D., P. H. Leiderman, C. R. Barnett, and J. A. Williams. "Effects of Mother-Infant Separation on Maternal Attachment Behavior." *Child Development*, 1972.

Loft, Kurt. "The Mozart Effect; Classical music, and Mozart in particular, could be a key in stimulating the mind to higher levels of reason, relaxation and creativity." *Tampa Tribune* February 20, 1998.

Macaulay, Lord. *Lays of Ancient Rome*. Washington DC: Gateway Books, 1997 ed.

Medved, Michael and Diane Medved, Ph.D. *Saving Childhood*. HarperCollins/Zondervan, 1998.

Miller, J. *The Body in Question*. N.Y.: Random House, 1978.

Montagu, A. "Animadversions on the Development of a Theory of Touch." *Touch in Early Development*, T. M. Field, ed. Mahwah, N.J.: Lawrence Erlbaum Associates, 1995.

Montagu, A. *Touching. The Human Significance of the Skin*. N.Y.: Harper & Row, 1971, p. 72.

Powell, L. F. "The Effect of Extra Stimulation and Maternal Involvement on the Development of Low-Birth-Weight Infants and on Maternal Behavior." *Child Development*, 1974.

Ribble, M. A. Disorganizing Factors of Infant Personality. *American Journal of Psychiatry*, 1941.

Rauscher, Frances H., Gordon L. Shaw, and Katherine N. Ky, "Music and Spatial Task Performance," *Nature*, 365 (1993): 611.

"The Riddle of the Mozart Effect; Music Therapy for Illness Care and Prevention." *Natural Health* January 11, 1998.

Newcomb. "Music Training Causes Long-term Enhancement of Preschool Children's Spatial-Temporal Reasoning," *Neurological Research* 19, 1997.

Schaefer, M., R.P. Hatcher, and P. D. Barglow. "Prematurity and Infant Stimulation: A Review of Research." *Child Psychiatry and Human Development*, 1980.

Solkoff, N. and D. Matuszak. Tactile Stimulation and Behavioral Development among Low-Birth weight Infants. *Child Psychiatry and Human Development*, 1975.

Stern, D. *The First Relationship. Mother and Infant*. Cambridge, Mass.: Harvard University Press, 1977.

Sutcliffe, Jenny, Dr., *Baby Bonding*. London: Virgin, 1994.

Tortora, G. and N. Anagnostakos. *Principles of Anatomy and Physiology*. 5th ed. N.Y.: Harper and Row, 1987.

White, J. L. and R. C. Labarba. "The Effects of Tactile and Kinesthetic Stimulation on Neonatal Development in the Premature Infant." *Developmental Psychobiology*, 1976.

RESOURCES/ADDRESSES

Brain Development:

Frank Porter Graham Child Development Center Chapel Hill, NC.

"Harper's Growing Tree" book series for infant/toddler brain development.

"So Smart" video by The Baby School Company (30 minutes, $14.95) (800) 663–2741.

"Baby's 1st Video," MVP Home Entertainment (30 minutes, $9.95). (800) 637–3555.

Breastfeeding:

La Leche League International (800) LA–LECHE.

Infant Massage:

Drehobl, K. F. and Fuhr, M. G. *Pediatric Massage for the Child with Special Needs.* Tucson, Arizona: Therapy Skill Builders, 1991. If you cannot find a copy of this book in your library, contact Communication Skill Builders, P.O. Box 42050, Tucson, Arizona 85733, (602) 323-7500.

International Association of Infant Massage Instructors (IAIMI) P.O. Box 438 Elma, New York 14059 (716) 652-9789.

The Loving Touch Cradle Care, Inc. PO Box 401548 Dallas, TX 75240 $20.00 for audio tape and illustrated instructions.

Sinclair, Marybetts. *Massage for Healthier Children.* Oakland, Calif.: Wingbow Press, 1992.

Kangaroo Care:

Dr. Susan Ludington University of Maryland at Baltimore School of Nursing Department of Maternal and Child Health 655 W. Lombard St. Baltimore, Maryland, 21201-1579 (send a stamped, self addressed envelope for a list of hospitals that provide Kangaroo Care).

Nutrition:

National Center for Nutrition and Dietetics Consumer Hotline (800) 638–2772.

Pregnancy/Women's Health

The American College of Obstetricians and Gynecologists (ACOG) Resource Center 409 12th Street SW Washington, DC 20024–2118 (202) 638–5577.

Maternal and Child Health Center (202) 625–8410.

Prenatal and Infant Learning:

BabyPlus UK Ltd 1–7 Harley Street London W1N 1DA 0171 637 1828.

The Children's Group Inc. classical music for children, babies, and unborn babies) 1400 Bayly Street, Ste. 7 Pickering, ON L1W 3R2 Canada (800) 757-8372 or (905) 831-1995 fax: (905) 831-1142 email: moreinfo@childrensgroup.com website: http://www.childrens-group.com

Heartsongs: Infants and Parents Sharing Music by Leon Thurman and Anna Peter Langness. Music Study Services PO Box 4665 Englewood, CO 80155 $14.95 plus postage and handling (audio tape and booklet)

The Infant Learning Company P.O. Box 189 Bonsall, CA 92003 1-888-READ-888 website: http://www.infantlearning.com

The Mozart Effect Resource Center 3526 Washington Avenue St. Louis, MO 63103-1019 800-721-2177 fax: 314-531-8384 website: music@mozarteffect.com

The Prenatal University by Dr. F. Rene Van de Carr The Prenatal University 27225 Calaroga Avenue Hayward, CA 94545

Sound Therapy:

Sound Healers Association Boulder, Colorado (303) 443-8181.

Touch:

Tiffany M. Field, Ph.D. Director, Touch Research Institute Department of Pediatrics (D-820) University of Miami School of Medicine P.O. Box 016820 Miami, Florida 33101 (305) 243-6781 or (305) 243-6790.

Vegetarianism:

Vegetarian Resource Group (410) 366–VEGE.

INDEX

A

abdomen, 31, 37–39, 58–59
abused children, 4, 11
acetylcholine, 155
Adderly Method of Infant Therapeutic Massage, 2, 3, 19, 21, 26–29
adoption, 8
aerobics, 52–55
aggression, 148
alcohol, 87, 88
alertness, 11
alphabet, 106–131
antioxidant, 155
apnea, 15, 18, 155
appetite, 17
arms and hands, 41–44, 54–55
aromatherapy, 23–25, 155
Asclepiades, 24
aspartame, 87
attachment behavior, 155
Auckett, Amelia, 6
axonal process, 12
ayurveda, 23, 156

B

back, 30–32, 49–51, 59
backpacks, 15
bath, 22, 66
blood, 18
body language, 62
bonding, parent-child, 1, 4, 15, 63–64, 156
bottle-feeding, 17
bradycardia, 156
brain, 1, 80–82, 84, 159
breastfeeding, 14, 83
bruises, 27

C

caffeine, 87–88
calendula, 86
Campbell, Don, 72
cardiac response, 8
Caribbean Primate Research Center, 150
cats, 152
chamomile, 86
child care, 71
chinese massage, 23
Chopra, Dr. Deepak, 152
circulation, 42, 46
colic, 57–59
conception, 79
congestion, 59–60
coordination, 14, 94
corticoid, 157
cortisol, 11, 16, 157
crying, 6
cytotoxicity, 157

D

dendritic processes, 9, 12
Denenberg, Dr. Victor, 147
Depardieu, Gerard, 70
dependency, 5
depression, 149
development, physical, 14, 79–82, 84, 91–103
diet, 83
digestion, 157
discomfort, 57
dogs, 152
dolphins, 152–53
drugs, 1, 11, 18–19, 88–89

E

ears, 35
echinacea, 86
electric shock, 152
empathy, 3
endorphins, 4
environment, 26–27
exercise, 15, 65
eye contact, 28

F

fat, 84
fetal position, 14, 158, 163
fetus, 12, 71, 77, 81
Field, Tiffany, Ph.D., 11
flexion, *see* fetal position
folic acid, 84
foods, 6, 80
foster homes, 8
Fox, Dr. Michael, 153

G

garlic, 86
genetics, 147
Greeks, massage and, 23–24
gregorian chant, 72

H

Hammett, Fredrick, 146
hands, importance of, 44
happiness, 2
head massage, 33–36
Heinrich, Steven, 152
herbs, 86–87
Herodicus, 24
Hindu, 23

Hippocrates, 23, 24
Holt, Dr. Luther E., 5
hormones, 19
horses, 152
hospitals, 7–8
hypochondria, 5
hypothalamus, 9

I

immune system, 149–50, 159
imprinting, 159
Indian massage, 29, 42
injuries, 64
intelligence quotient, 8, 69, 84, 85
International Association of Infant Massage, 64
iron, 84
isolation, 148

K

Kangaroo Care, 11–14
Kennell, John, 10
kinesthetic stimulation, 17
Klaus, Marshall, 10

L

language, development of, 2, 28, 77, 93, 95, 134–43
legs and feet, 45–48, 52–53
Lilly, Dr. John, 152
Ling, Pehr Henrik, 24
love, expression of, 4
lymph system, 45
Lynch, Dr. James, 152

M

Mason, Dr. M. L., 146
massage: benefits to giver, 11, 26; history of, 23–25
maternal separation, 149, 150, 151
maternal-neonatal thermal synchrony, 15
mathematics, 2, 70
memory, 81, 94, 96
metacarpal bone, 19
Metzger, Dr., 25
Miller, Zell, 71
mint, 86
Montague, Dr. Ashley, 3
morning sickness, 24
MRI, 71
muscular coordination, 18
music, 2, 69, 73, 75
myuelination, 9

N

nervous system, 19, 70, 155, 161, 163
nicotine, 87
nissl bodies, 9, 161
numeral images, 134–43
nutrasweet, 87
nutrition, 2, 83–90

O

oil, 22–26, 37, 45, 49, 64
opera, 76, 77
oriental massage, 29
ornithine decarboxylase, 147
orphanages, 8
oxygen, 18

P

Pare, Ambroise, 24
parent, importance of, 19, 82, 92
percussion, 161
pets, massage of, 153–54
phenylalanine, 87
pigs, 145
Plato, 73
position for massage, 27, 162, 163
post-partum depression, 5
prayer, 77
pregnancy, 80, 89
premature babies, 7–10, 12, 16, 29, 159, 161
preschool children, 17, 67, 69
pressure, level of, 29
primates, 148

R

rabbits, 152
radius bone, 19
rats, 146–47
reading, 96–101
Reite, Dr. Martin, 149
relaxation, 15, 42, 46
respiratory problems, 17, 162
response from child, 27, 57
Rice Infant Sensorimotor Stimulation (RISS), 8, 15
Rice, Ruth Dianne, 8, 9
Romans, use of massage, 24
routine, importance of, 27, 28
Royal Touch, 24

S

schizophrenia, 149
self-confidence, 19, 28
serotonin, 4
sexual identity, 149
Shaw, Dr. Gordon, 70

INDEX

singing, 93
skin, 3, 27, 157, 158, 162
sleep, 15–17, 62, 149
smile, 28, 93
social behaviors, 3, 94, 150–51
somotrophin, 9
sonic healing, 72
speech, development of, 70, 91–92, 94
spine, 31, 32
Spitz, Dr. Rene A., 7, 146
starvation, of touch, 8
stimulation and overstimulation, 5, 17, 29, 91
stress, 19, 56
strokes, 158
subliminal learning, 95
Suomi, Dr. Stephen J., 150
swedish massage, 29, 42, 153
Swedish Movement Cure, 24–25

T

tachycardia, 163
talking, during massage, 28
taurine, 84
television, 102
Tellington-Jones, Linda, 153
therapy, 64, 148
thinking, conceptual, 2
thrive, failure to, 7–8
tibia bone, 19
toddlers, 56
Tomatis Center, 70
Tomatis, Alfred, 72
Touch Research Institute, 11, 16, 22
toxic culture, 102–103
toys, 92, 94
TTouch, 153

U

University of Konstanz, 71
University of Miami School of Medicine, 11, 16

V

vagus nerve, 4, 163
violence, 73, 102–103
vitamin B-12, 86
voice, mother's, 77, 79

W

Watson, Dr. John, 5
weaning, 6, 147, 163
weight, 12, 16, 85
Whimbey, Dr. Arthur, 147

Y

yoga, for babies, 9

Z

zinc, 84–85

A special thanks to
Miss Sidney Helen Burger

ORDER EXTRA COPIES FOR YOUR LOVED ONES!

BRIGHTER BABY

Boost Your Child's Intelligence, Health, & Happiness through Infant Therapeutic Massage, the Mozart Effect, and more...

by Jay Gordon, M.D. and Brenda Adderly, M.H.A.

How to increase your baby's intelligence, health, and happiness through touch

Brighter Baby, coauthored by Brenda Adderly and Dr. Jay Gordon, one of America's leading pediatricians, demonstrates how therapeutic baby massage—long known for its ability to improve bonding between parent and child—actually increases your baby's IQ and measurably improves his or her physical health.

In *Brighter Baby* parents will learn to help their child's early development through:

- Touch to stimulate appetite, wellness, and even their baby's capacity for learning
- Music and the "Mozart Effect" to encourage intellectual development
- Proper nutrition to give their baby the best possible head start in life
- And "brain exercises" to engage their child's mind

Brighter Baby gives parents all the necessary tools to prepare their child for the challenges of life.

Order direct and SAVE 20% PLUS free Priority Mail shipping!

BOOKSTORE PRICE $19.95
YOURS FOR ONLY $15.95

TO ORDER CALL 1-888-219-4747

Or send check or money order to:
LifeLine Press • P.O. Box 97199 • Washington DC 20090-7199
Be sure to mention code RSP134 when you call or write.

Become Your Child's Favorite Teacher!

Give your child the power of **CREATIVITY** and **CONCENTRATION** with two new books from PLAYSKOOL

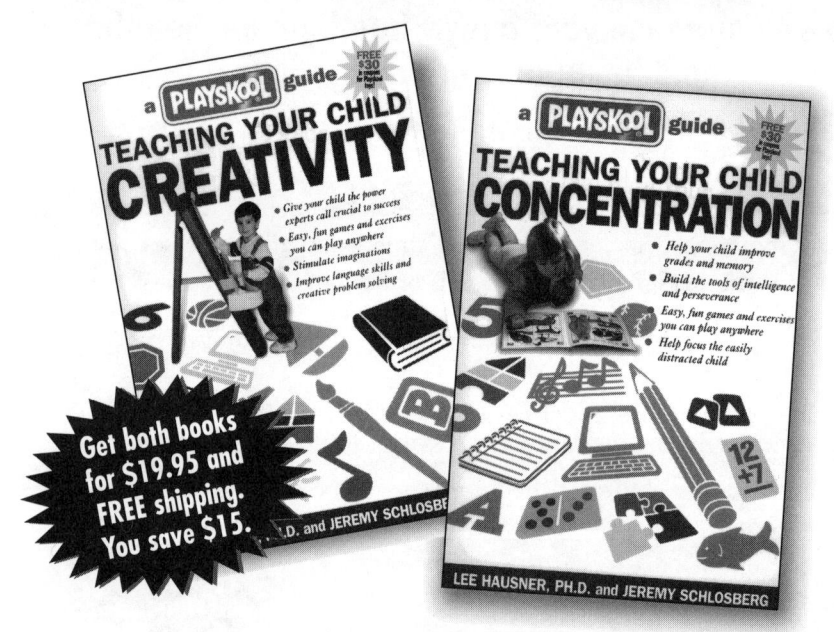

Get both books for $19.95 and FREE shipping. You save $15.

Extensive research shows creative and focused children achieve more and go on to lead happier, richer lives.

Without **CREATIVITY** or **CONCENTRATION**, even children with high IQs or good grades may not live up to their potential later in life. Now, the child development experts at PLAYSKOOL along with Dr. Lee Hausner, show how easy it is to actually "teach" your children these essential traits and how fun it can be to do so!

Now, with the purchase of these two books, you will become your child's favorite teacher and at the same time help give him or her a head start in school and in life. The games and activities presented here give your child the power to succeed!

The Playskool **CREATIVITY** and **CONCENTRATION** Guides show you how to:

- **Learn through play:** easy, fun games and exercises you can play anywhere with your child.

- **Stimulate imaginations** in children using the same creativity workshop concepts used by such business giants as AT&T, CBS, Coca-Cola, General Electric, and IBM.

> *"It's always such a delight to find books which really help children be the best they can be. This one fits the bill."*
> **—Dr. Joyce Brothers**

- **Improve** grades and memory skills with simple, mind-stimulating exercises and activities.

- **Expand** creativity and enhance concentration through storytelling and make-believe.

- **Teach** creative problem solving—a basic component of IQ.

- **Increase** your child's attention span and overcome the distractions of television and video games.

- **Create** a home environment that encourages ongoing learning.

- **Give your child the power to succeed.**

▼ Detach here and mail today ▼

Order now and you can have both books for only $19.95
(Regular price for both books would be almost $30! With FREE shipping you save $15).

Call 1-888-219-4747

Operators are available 24 hours.
Or, if you prefer, copy this coupon and mail it in an envelope with your payment as indicated below:

☐ **Yes,** please send me ____ sets of *Teaching Your Child Creativity* and *Teaching Your Child Concentration*.

  ☐ Enclosed is my check for $19.95 per set (includes expedited shipping and handling). Make check payable to LifeLine Press.
  or
  ☐ Charge my ☐ VISA ☐ MasterCard ☐ American Express ☐ DISCOVER

Name_____Phone_____
Street_____
City_____ State_____ Zip_____
Credit card #_____Exp.Date___/___
Signature_____

FOR PRIORITY SERVICE CALL 1-888-219-4747
Or mail order to: LifeLine Press. • P.O. Box 97199 • Washington, D.C. 20090-7199
(Fax orders to 202-216-0611)